THE COVID-19 PANDEMIC

Restarting In The New Era

Patricia I. Natpikia (PhD)

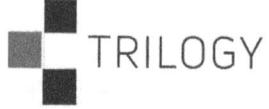

Trilogy Christian Publishers
A Wholly Owned Subsidiary of Trinity Broadcasting Network
2442 Michelle Drive
Tustin, CA 92780
Copyright © 2024 by Patricia I. Natpikia
Scripture quotations marked NIV are taken from the Holy Bible, New International Version®, NIV®. Copyright © 1973, 1978, 1984, 2011 by Biblica, Inc.TM Used by permission of Zondervan. All rights reserved worldwide. www.zondervan.com. The "NIV" and "New International Version" are trademarks registered in the United States Patent and Trademark Office by Biblica, Inc.TM. Scripture quotations marked NKJV are taken from the New King James Version®. Copyright © 1982 by Thomas Nelson. Used by permission. All rights reserved. Scripture quotations marked KJV are taken from the King James Version of the Bible. Public domain.
All rights reserved, including the right to reproduce this book or portions thereof in any form whatsoever.
For information, address Trilogy Christian Publishing
Rights Department, 2442 Michelle Drive, Tustin, Ca 92780.
Trilogy Christian Publishing/ TBN and colophon are trademarks of Trinity Broadcasting Network.
For information about special discounts for bulk purchases, please contact Trilogy Christian Publishing.
Trilogy Disclaimer: The views and content expressed in this book are those of the author and may not necessarily reflect the views and doctrine of Trilogy Christian Publishing or the Trinity Broadcasting Network.
10 9 8 7 6 5 4 3 2 1
Library of Congress Cataloging-in-Publication Data is available.
ISBN 979-8-89333-315-2
ISBN 979-8-89333-316-9 (ebook)

DEDICATION

This book is dedicated to the sweet memories of yesteryears. To the days and months lost to the pandemic and to a blissful tomorrow filled with hope and gladness through faith.

ACKNOWLEDGMENTS

The support, encouragement, and contributions received in the creation of this book are enormous and not in any way taken for granted. Without these, this book could not have been created. I acknowledge everyone. Permit me, however, to mention but a few.

First and foremost, I give thanks to God Almighty, who calls according to His purpose and for the glorification of His name. He who makes a way where there seems to be no way to refresh and sustain us. To Him be all glory, honor, and adoration.

To my numerous interviewees, clients, friends, and colleagues who gave this project not just their time and attention but their hearts and souls as well, I am highly indebted. Without any limitations, they shared their stories and experiences, which I found very informative and inspiring enough to include in this book. I say a big thank you to you all.

To all first-ponderers: the healthcare workers (active and retired), paramedics, clergies, fire and rescue workers, for your indelible services during the pandemic. You are all highly acknowledged and appreciated.

To spouses, partners, and family members who stood in for their absentee pandemic heroes during their call to duty, you are all highly recognized.

To my publisher, I am eternally indebted and say thank you for re-directing my thoughts and helping my dream and purpose come alive.

To those numerous men and women who live and remain in faith in Christ and in the power of His words and promises, thereby walking in victory, proving God's ability to do exceedingly abundantly above all we ask or think. I salute you all.

To my wonderful family, who has given me love and support throughout this project, I say thank you for always believing in me and in the importance of this project. God Almighty bless you all.

TABLE OF CONTENTS

Preface 11
Introduction 13
Chapter 1: Exploring the Fear of Change 21
    The Pandemic Timeline 23
    A Trip Down Memory Lane 25
    A Whole New World 27

Chapter 2: Exploring the Pandemic-Altered Society 31
    The Evolution of a Pandemic-Altered Society 33
    Turning the Focus to Mental Health 35
    Pandemic Heroes 37
    Working Remotely 39
    Overview of an Altered Pandemic Society 41
    The End of the Pandemic 43

Chapter 3: Exploring the Struggles of Adjusting to the Whole New World 47
    The Meaning of Life—Through the Eyes of
    Pandemic Warriors 50
    Exploring the Meaning of Life in a Pandemic World 51
    Facing Challenges During the Search for the Meaning
    of Life 53
    Find Your Meaning of Life 55

Chapter 4: Utilizing the Voice of Reason to Embrace Changes 57
    Implementing Tools to Cope with Change 59
    Breaking the Fear of Normal Barriers 60
    Erring on the Side of Worry 61
    Introducing Positivity 63
    Learning How to Cope with Change 65
    The Stages of Change 67
    You Are Stronger than You Think 68

Chapter 5: Adjusting to Your New Workplace in the Pandemic-Altered World 71
    Working from Home 73
    Making Sweet Lemonade Out of Sour Lemons 74
    Scheduling 75
    Appropriate Workspace 76
    Rise and Shine 77
    Facing Challenges 77
    Setting Yourself up for Success 78
        Comfortable Work Chair 79
        Keyboard Setup 79
        Essential Office Tools 79
    Additional Measures to Succeed When Working Remotely 80
    Adapting to the New Dynamics in the Workplace 81
    Introducing Workplace Models 83
        The Old New Normal Model 84
        The Hybrid Model 84
        Jack-in-the-Box Model 84
        The Satellite Office Model 85
        Virtual Reality Model 86
    Adopting Workplace Dynamics for the Future 86
    The Benefits of the Hybrid Model 87

    Connecting Technology and Humans 88
    A Gig-Based Employment Market.............................. 88
    Real-Life Adjustments 89

Chapter 6: Putting the Pieces of Your Pandemic-Altered Work Life Back Together 93
    Easing Your Way Back to Working at the Office 96
    Adjusting to Your Brand-New Normal Work-Life 98
    The Art of Compassion 100
    Establishing New Routines.. 100
    Setting Boundaries in the Workplace 101
    Learning How to Create a Healthy Work-
    Life Balance.. 101
    Understanding Work-Life Balance.............................. 102
    Job Hunting in A Pandemic-Altered World 105
    Free Courses 107
    Volunteering... 107

Chapter 7: Financial Insecurity in Your Pandemic-Altered World 111
    Your Journey to Financial Health and Well-Being 113
    A Glimpse into the Financial Future of a
    World in Crisis 114
    Spending and Saving Habits During a
    Global Pandemic.. 116
    Financial Hits and Misses.. 117
    Spending Money During a Pandemic 118
    Re-Evaluating Your Personal Financial Habits 119
    Habits for Consideration... 121
        Debt Busting 121
        Savings One-Oh-One 122
        The Thrice-Turned Dollar 122
        A Little 123
    Examples of Implementing New Habits 123

Creating Your Breaking-Free Budget 124
Commuting Woes 126
Lunch Time 126
Caffeine Fix 127
What about the Children? 127
Final Round-Up 128
Conclusion 130
No More Hiding Behind the Pandemic 131
The Final Word 133

About the Author 135

References 137

PREFACE

Many are the struggles that come with adjusting and coping with life after a long shutdown, such as with the COVID-19 pandemic, which took the entire world by surprise. There are the new setups that give anxiety and pressure, the many life disruptions that come in so many ways, not knowing how to adjust to the new lifestyle, and the other desires of some to learn ways to improve themselves. All these challenges, and many more, must be contended with.

This book gives answers to many of these concerns. It introduces readers to a guide that teaches how to adjust to the new normal of post-pandemic life. Applying real-life examples, the author methodologically explores various social, emotional, economic, and psychological perspectives, looking at each of them along with tips and strategies to ensure readers can restart their lives and live healthily and happily. The beauty and benefits of living in the truth of the Lord who forgives all iniquities, heals all diseases, redeems life from destruction, crowns with loving kindness and tender mercies, and satisfies our mouth with good things so that our youth is renewed like the eagle's are found to be fundamental to the entire transformation process.

INTRODUCTION

"The human capacity for burden is like bamboo—far more flexible than you'd ever believe at first glance" (Jodi Picoult).

COVID-19 will always be known as the pandemic that brought the globe to a screeching halt and flipped the world upside down. The population watched and listened to the news as the continents shared the details of what was happening in their respective countries. People kept a very close eye on the statistics that featured those who had been infected, admitted to hospitals, and the death tolls. Fear spread like wildfire, which saw individuals flocking to the stores to stock up on food and whatever they felt they needed. It wasn't very long before the respective heads of state and governments announced that schools, places of worship, fitness centers, and any activities that involved gatherings were being stopped until further notice. It was a difficult time for many, and the idea of being confined to their homes may have seemed like a fun idea, but the tables were turned when the four walls started closing in.

The reality is that many had to live with the restrictions that were imposed by the various countries. Imagine living in a country where the ocean is your backyard, and you are being told that you may not sit on the beach and enjoy the natural vitamin D boosters. Imagine being forcefully removed from the beach by law enforcement officers because you are breaking the rules. This is the reality that countries faced during the stay-at-home or lock-down orders set out by governments.

I heard of a country putting a ban on the purchase of alcohol and cigarettes for nearly nine months to force individuals to stay out of stores. The government believed that they were winning, only to discover that bootlegging became a lucrative (and tax-avoidance) business that defied the purpose of the lock-down orders.

Religious gatherings and other traditional communal worshiping were restrained. Churches closed their doors in response to the directives, and some created an innovative way to stay connected through virtual prayer meetings. When restrictions finally allowed, many shifted to on-line services, while others implemented safely measures such as social distancing and mask-wearing for in-person gatherings. Other essential workers worked remotely from their homes. It was a trying period for all.

Lizzy, a seventy-nine-year-old grandmother of five, later told of how many challenges she faced adapting to virtual worship. She confessed missing the sense of community and connection she had felt during in-person gatherings. She joined the group of members who struggled with the technology relating to virtual worship.

Family members and friends were lost to the pandemic. While many struggled with feelings of loss, grief, and anger, others grappled with a range of emotions and questions. Amid it all, only faith in the power of God's words and promises spoke for many. It served as a cushion and source of strength and hope, confessed a middle-aged lady whose husband of eighteen years and father of their four young children was infected and in a coma for almost eight weeks. In her words, "At my lowest period, I called to remembrance my faith in the power in the Word and promises of God. His promises are numerous and effective, and my shame and pain were taken away. I was given beauty for ashes, a garment of praise for heaviness" (Isaiah 61:3).

Governments and health organizations implemented strong surveillance systems, quick response protocols, and improved healthcare infrastructure to better manage future outbreaks. The society also saw ongoing emphasis on vaccination campaigns, public health measures, and research into treatment and preventives. In the entire period, the redeemed of the Lord remained in faith, hope, and trust in the Lord. The instructions of the Lord are perfect; they revive the soul; the decrees are trustworthy, making wise the simple; the commandments are right, bringing joy to the heart; the commands are clear, giving insight for living; the laws are true, each one is fair; they are more desirable than gold even the finest gold. They are sweeter than honey, even honey dripping from the comb (Psalm 19:7–10). Not everyone takes advantage of this incredible source of strength. Too often, we view God's words and promises through the lens of others, distorted, darkened, and shattered.

The Reality of Living in a Pandemic

I do believe that it is safe to assume that we all relied on mainstream media coverage to keep us in the loop of what was going on in our communities, countries, and in the rest of the world. I will be the first to admit that a lot of the media coverage was upsetting to me, and I suspect that I am not the only person who was affected by the visuals that we got to see on our screens.

Many individuals were embraced by fear instead of reassurance because it was something that the world had never dealt with before. We were entering new territories, and people were afraid, traumatized, and didn't know what to think.

The World Health Organization (WHO) noted that the first year of the pandemic saw an overall increase of 25 percent across the globe for individuals struggling with mental health conditions such as depression and anxiety (2022). It was further noted that this global increase was only the beginning, as it was affecting all people across all walks of life. Mental health has no boundaries and doesn't discriminate against anyone. It will always rear its head to break individuals down.

Year two of the pandemic saw many changes to accommodate our new way of life and living. Many of the countries started easing restrictions; some even flung the doors wide open to announce that all restrictions were abolished, and others kept many of their draconian laws with slight modifications.

Mental Health America (MHA) provided a platform where individuals could participate in online mental health screenings. More than 5.4 million people participated in these screenings in 2021. It is believed that youngsters between the ages of eleven to seventeen made up 45 percent of the individuals who were screened and identified with mental health concerns. An alarming 76 percent of Americans—adults and youth—suffer from emotional and behavioral problems, have anxiety, or are triggered by the effects of trauma ("Mental Health and COVID-19," n.d.).

I know what it's like to feel ugly inside, alone, afraid, and broken. I have been there. You will see me express my faith as you read on because I have had my share of the experience; I have discovered the balm. We often limit the Lord in the affairs of our lives when we lack the faith to rest on the power of His words and promises. "Those who know your name trust in you, for you, LORD, have never forsaken those who seek You" (Psalm 9:10, NIV).

Year three of the pandemic life is a little different than the days of all the restrictions. We have a lot more freedom to live life to the fullest, but I have experienced that people are still holding onto some fear. The media coverage, although limited, still talks about various strains of the virus, and you hear—via a couple of grapevines—that this one has got COVID-19 and that another one is getting over it. Many people have asked if COVID-19 will ever be eradicated, and that is a question no one has an answer to. You do have conspiracy theorists who will be loud and proud in saying that COVID-19 is not real and that everything connected to it is a scare-mongering tactic from governments across the world. I don't entertain conspiracy theories, but I do believe that the individuals hiding behind the masks are looking for answers.

A Glimpse into the Struggles of the Pandemic

I believe that the COVID-19 pandemic was nature's way of slowing the world down. We are always in a rush to get from point A to Z, so we don't pay attention to what goes on between the two points. The first couple of months of the stay-home orders saw the rivers, lakes, oceans, forests, and general nature find healing. The pandemic allowed the earth to heal, take a breath, and enjoy some of the freedom it had forgotten existed. The pandemic may have given nature a slight reprieve, but it did come at the expense of the lives and health of innocent people who were infected. The COVID-19 virus brought more baggage on its vacation than anyone could ever have anticipated. No one really expects a "vacation" to last longer than two years, but here we are—still playing host to a virus that changed and continues to change the lives of billions of people.

One of the most devastating effects of the pandemic, other than the loss of lives and the permanent effects of the virus, is that people lost their means to support themselves or their families. The financial strain on individuals contributed to their resentment because of the constant worry about where the next meal would come from and how they would keep a roof over their heads, water flowing through their taps, or power to keep them warm. Many people turned to charitable organizations for support and felt that their pride had been tarnished because they were asking instead of assisting.

I have found that a lot of my interviewees have built up a lot of anger toward the pandemic in general. It would be easy to point fingers and lay blame on the government and those individuals who ignored the mandates or even be angry at themselves. At the end of a very long day, we need to realize that no amount of blame is going to be a remedy for what has happened. This was new territory to all of us, and no amount of preparation could have prepared us for what was to come. We can blame the government or even the WHO, but the point of the matter is that they, too, were treading in dark and murky waters. You didn't know what was going on or what was going to happen. You may have been one of those who graduated from the University of Google Medical Center and gained your PhD in Couch Surfing during this time—no judgment because you would not be the first, and certainly not the last.

Sharing her story with a group at a mid-week worship service, Maria, a mother of six, attributed her family's survival of the financial constraints and hardship to the generosity of the community and her faith in divine provision (Philippians 4:19). In her words, "It was impossible not being anxious when you have eight hungry mouths to feed, but I had to learn to practice what I always taught: patience, trust, and in everything by prayer and supplication with thanksgiving let your request be made known to God. Just like Elijah got fed by ravens in the cave in Cherith (1 Kings 17:3). Help came, and people kept coming to share with us." This is only one of the many stories of how people fought to live above the torturous waters of the pandemic.

Adapting to the New Normal

I recently learned that many people view change as being the enemy. They would prefer to keep everything the same and add in bits and pieces without any major changes. Can I tell you a secret? Change is not the enemy, and it is something that everyone should embrace. Changes are scary, but they open a set of doors that lead you to new experiences. I have always been a huge advocate for having an open mind, living in the present, and embracing all the big and little changes that form part of your journey through life. A renewal of the mind (Romans 12:2). Do not overreact or overplay the impact. Accept that changes in life are natural and often inevitable.

The new normal involves a lot more than adapting and implementing changes; it also involves your mental health. I get angry when I hear the uninformed say that people will snap out of their state of depression as soon as the pandemic is over. Who says the pandemic will ever be over? Who knows how long COVID-19 will boomerang on innocent people for four, five, or six years after the onset? The future is uncertain, and the pandemic didn't come with an expiration date. Let us leave for God the future, which is uncertain. The restrictions may have been eased, and we may be embracing our new normal, but we will never forget that the pandemic exists. All that has happened is that we have adapted our lives to be vigilant and continue practicing safety measures that include washing our hands, embracing general health protocols, such as coughing and sneezing into our arms, and staying away from events if we are feeling unwell. We will not be anxious about anything.

> **Be anxious for nothing, but in everything by prayer and supplication, with thanksgiving, let your requests be made known to God; and the peace of God, which surpasses all understanding, will guard your hearts and minds through Christ Jesus.**
>
> Philippians 4:6–7 (NKJV)

We are adapting to the new normal. This is the reason why I am writing this book. I want to help individuals avoid the point where they feel they have nowhere to go. This book is your safe place, and I will remind you of this throughout this book. You will not be judged, bullied, or condemned for your thoughts or actions. No one in this book cares about your ethnicity, religion, financial standing, or your career because—here—you are protected. Let's put on some comfortable leisurewear, fill that Stanley cup with pebble ice, grab some treats, and explore this journey of the new normal.

CHAPTER 1:
Exploring the Fear of Change

"Be ye transformed by the renewing of your mind, that ye may prove what is that good, and acceptable, and perfect"

(Romans 12:2, KJV).

"For the Spirit God gave us does not make us timid"

(2 Timothy 1:7, NIV).

"Don't be afraid of change. You may lose something, but you may gain something better" (anonymous).

I have previously touched on the fact that people may be afraid of change, especially when suddenly introduced and immediately put into effect. I think of the elderly who are set in their ways and have a rock-solid routine that they follow from the moment they wake up until they go to bed. To force an elderly person to implement changes at this later stage of their lives would be traumatic to them. I have also found that many individuals do not cope well with sudden changes because they have established a routine that helps them remain grounded.

No one could have foreseen that a pandemic would spread like wildfire through the continents, claim lives, and threaten the health of innocent victims. No one could have predicted that our lives, as we knew them, would be restricted to six feet apart human interaction and wearing masks. We had to adapt, whether we wanted to or not, to the changes that were imposed upon us by the respective governing bodies of the different countries, states, or counties.

I recall witnessing an interaction between two people at the store one day. One of the ladies was well into her nineties, and the other in her late forties, and they were well-acquainted because of family friends. The new COVID-19 store was set up to replicate a racecourse to ensure that everyone stayed in their lanes and six feet apart. The elderly lady saw her young friend and broke the rules to go and hug her, as onlookers gasped in shock.

The elderly lady was not on board with the changes imposed on her, and she wasn't going to let anyone tell her any different. She understood the risks of closing the distance of that six-feet-apart rule, but as she explained to the store owner who told her that his license was at risk, "I'm an old lady who is not used to being forced to sit in a box without showing my friends how much I care about them. This friend needed a hug; her eyes told me, and I can't ignore the call of the eyes."

I have found that the older generation did have a tough time adjusting to and adopting the changes that were meant to be beneficial to their physical health. The story of the elderly lady is proof that they may be told what to do but that they won't be okay with the directions they are given. I have previously mentioned that the COVID-19 pandemic didn't give anyone time to get used to the idea of changes; many of those changes happened overnight, and others had a week or two to prepare.

The Pandemic Timeline

We were introduced to the statistics and heartbreaking news of the effects of the pandemic as it was happening in real-time. I don't think that we ever envisioned that the severity of the effects of the pandemic would reach our country or even our cities. I believe that many people may have believed that they were protected and untouchable. It would come as a shock to many that no one was immune to the effects of the pandemic. But for the faith in divine intervention (Psalm 3:3).

It was up to every household to make the changes that would keep them as protected from the virus as possible. That would mean that the children couldn't go to friends' houses or that families couldn't pop in for a visit. Work and school looked different for everyone. Children shifted to online schooling, and parents had to supervise that everyone was doing their daily lessons. The dynamics for the working sector changed, and home offices were being set up so that people could work remotely—after all, the show must go on.

Not everyone was given the opportunity to work remotely or have online schooling. These changes in dynamics were detrimental to the mental health and well-being of millions of individuals. These individuals may have been working in construction, as tellers or line cooks at fast-food restaurants, or as salespeople before the rug was pulled out from under them. These are people who live paycheck-to-paycheck to keep food on their tables and a roof over their heads. I can almost guarantee that these individuals will tell you that, while they don't have much, they get by on love, faith, and hope. The bottom line is that everyone—regardless of their work situation, their income, or their social standing—has had to adapt to the changes imposed by the COVID-19 pandemic restrictions.

We may be three years into this pandemic, but I do believe that many people are still subconsciously following some of the restrictions—minus the face masks. Remember that I am not here to tell you how to live your life or what you should be doing. I am writing this book from an observer's point of view and using information that I have picked up from interviewing my clients and colleagues. I know that a lot of what will be said will be triggering and bring up some painful memories, but it is not my intention to add to anyone's trauma. It is important to your mental health to face the triggers that you have been exposed to over the last couple of years to learn to appreciate and express your source of strength.

We can't do anything about the past; it happened, it left its mark, and we've adjusted as best we could. It is essential to go back to the beginning of the timeline and understand the turn of events that led us to where we find ourselves in 2023 and beyond. Remember that you don't have to be afraid of what

Chapter 1: Exploring the Fear of Change

has happened because it can't hurt you anymore. The only way forward is to look to the present and the future (Psalm 130:7).

A Trip Down Memory Lane

I stumbled across a website by the name of Think Global Health and came across some interesting information. As of February 24, 2023, the total global number of confirmed Coronavirus cases is a whopping 647,809,997. These are individuals who have been confirmed to have been infected since the outbreak of the pandemic in 2019. The total global number of deaths stands at 6,868,946 people (Kantis et al., n.d.). Our hearts go out to the families, friends, and loved ones who suffered—and who may still suffer—losses. This reaffirms something that I tell my friends, family, colleagues, and clients: Life is not guaranteed except eternal life, which is granted in the promises in John 10:28 (KJV), "And I give unto them eternal life; and they shall never perish, neither shall any man pluck them out of my hand."

I know and understand that the pandemic has been the topic of many heated discussions. Many heads have been butted because everyone has an opinion that they believe to be their truth. Graduates from the University of Google Medical Center have put their PhD in Couch Surfing to excellent use. These are the people we want to avoid at all costs because they are getting their information from sources that have not been verified. They continue to spread fear and incite hate because, in my opinion, they are afraid to step out of the bubbles that they have created for themselves.

Let's look at the timeline that got us to where we find ourselves today. It is important to remember that we are not going to be pointing fingers or spreading any hate towards countries or individuals. You can't change what has already happened, and that is why you are on this journey. You will identify areas on the timeline where you started to experience that shift in your life.

December 2019.

- Chinese health officials treated patients for an unknown illness in Wuhan. Days later, it was announced that the patients had tested positive for the Coronavirus.

January 2020.

- The Coronavirus claimed its first victim in Wuhan. The virus spread to other countries such as Japan, South Korea, and the United States. Chinese authorities intervened and locked down Wuhan.
- The World Health Organization announced that the world may be facing a health emergency.
- The United States enforced a travel ban on China.

February 2020.

- The WHO named the virus "COVID-19."
- This month saw an increase in deaths in many countries, such as France, the United States, Brazil, and Italy.

March 2020.

- Mandates and restrictions came into effect, with the Centers for Disease Control and Prevention (CDC) recommending limitations on in-person gatherings for American citizens.
- The European Union imposed travel restrictions outside of its territories.
- India and other countries announced lockdowns starting with twenty-one days and being adjusted as governments see fit.

Chapter 1: Exploring the Fear of Change

April 2020.

- Job losses continued to increase, with the New York Times alluding that more than ten million jobs had been lost in mere weeks of the outbreak of the pandemic (Taylor, 2021).
- A mask mandate was imposed on all travelers and flight attendants.

The present-day COVID-19 timeline continues with information about new strains of the virus emerging, borders opening after travel bans, or vaccines being administered. The vaccine is a sore point, which I do not feel should be a focal point of this book. I do believe that everyone should choose without being pressured. It is a personal choice, and no one should tell or make you feel otherwise. I would request that my readers be respectful when leaving comments and that everyone refrain from bullying or condemnation.

A Whole New World

It is safe to say that the global pandemic introduced changes that most people may not have adopted had it not been enforced. It is difficult to alter habits that you may have had in place for many years. I know that the older generation has created comfort zones for themselves and only applied minimal changes to keep up with the demands of life. No one could have foreseen that a global pandemic would infiltrate our lives and force us to change age-old habits that kick us out of our comfort zones.

The changes that were imposed caused fear, panic, and anxiety because everyone was uncertain about what was happening. Mainstream media outlets—and messages from the WHO, the CDC, and government officials—didn't take the time to explain the finer details to help people understand what was happening.

We must remember that not everyone is technologically savvy, nor do they understand why things must change. I have spoken to many people from all walks of life who have expressed their opinions regarding the lack of communication and failure to help people understand what was happening.

I find myself looking back at the first couple of months when stay-at-home or lock-down orders were imposed. The tides had changed for everyone because it was something that no one had ever been forced to do before the global pandemic swept across the world. That novelty wore off eventually, and people started to push the boundaries because they wanted to go out and see friends or have a cup of coffee at a local coffee shop. The moment the novelty started wearing off was when the new world was created. This was when we realized that, going forward, changes needed to be adopted and recognized because we had a new resident who wasn't planning on leaving in a hurry. For many others, it was a time to reaffirm their trust in the supernatural protection of the Lord. In ignorance, there is no victory for the believer. You must take responsibility to establish superior spiritual illumination.

The strain of accommodating this new resident has affected the mental health of billions of individuals across the globe. Many are and have been receiving the help they need, but then, you have people who are afraid or ashamed to seek professional help. These individuals are afraid of being judged, bullied, or condemned for their "weaknesses" and would prefer to suffer in silence. These are the people we need to reach out to and get them the help that they need.

It is not a secret that the arrival of the pandemic plunged the global population into a state of confusion. No one knew what the future would look like. Let's take a giant step into chapter

2 to discover how the pandemic opened a portal that embraced changes, recognized unsung heroes, and offered solutions to keep thriving during the hard times. Let's continue our journey and uncover some of the treasures the new world has put on display. Are we ready?

CHAPTER 2:

Exploring the Pandemic-Altered Society

"You never change things by fighting the existing reality. To change something, build a new model that makes the existing model obsolete"

(R. Buckminster Fuller).

News about COVID-19 filtered in through mainstream media and social media at the end of 2019. Everyone became focused on what a global pandemic would mean to their lives and lifestyles. Not many seemed to notice that, in addition to the pandemic, the world was being plagued by a host of natural disasters. I remember telling friends that COVID-19 didn't only bring a pandemic but that it brought devastating consequences to harm our ecosystem. These natural disasters added to the anxiety of individuals because many were left destitute, the land was destroyed, and plagues joined the pandemic.

Australia found itself battling a bushfire that claimed the lives of innocent people, the loss of over 5,900 homes and businesses, and damage to approximately 46 million acres (18.6 million hectares) of ground. A flood in Indonesia claimed the lives of even more innocent people who either drowned in the floods, were dragged under the water by landslides, or were shocked by electrical wires. The Philippines saw a volcano erupt after forty-six years of being dormant, as well as a volcano-tectonic earthquake that shook the country to its core.

The first half of 2020 saw many natural disasters that were uncommon but not unheard of. Internet sleuths believed that the world had entered the end of times despite biblical teachings on this; religious fundamentalists had a field day, gathering all their proof and preparing for the second coming (Monteiro, 2020).

I had to step outside of the conspiracy bubble to take stock of all the information I had gathered. The pandemic swooped into our lives like a thief in the night. There was nothing much anyone could do but follow protocol as presented by government officials and organizations. The natural disasters had me frowning as I tried to understand what was happening. It then dawned on me that the only reason these natural disasters are standing out is that we are paying attention to what is going on outside of our comfort bubbles. The world slowed down because of the pandemic, and we had more time to see what was happening in other countries. The last couple of years have seen the world go through a lot of turmoil, where we saw neighboring countries declare war on each other, earthquakes tearing through Turkey and Syria, and extreme weather conditions sweeping through North America. This is not, however, to say that we have not been warned that nations shall rise against nations, and kingdom against kingdom: and there shall be earthquakes in divers places, and there shall be famines and troubles (Mark 13:8, KJV). Those who trust in the Lord have a hiding place. As David cried, I will take refuge in the shadow of Your wings until these calamities have passed by. I will cry out to You, God, who performs all things for me.

Have mercy on me, my God, have mercy on me, for in you I take refuge. I will take refuge in the shadow of your wings until the disaster has passed. I cry out to God Most High, to God, who vindicates me.

Psalm 57:1–2 (NIV)

The Evolution of a Pandemic-Altered Society

World leaders joined forces with their counterparts, consulted various health organizations, and came up with a plan of action to curb the spread of the virus. Some countries were a little overbearing and harsh with their restrictions, which resulted in people pushing boundaries. Other countries were accused of being too lax. The Google PhD graduates took to forums and social media platforms and approached whoever they could think of to spread their truths about the COVID-19 pandemic. Everyone had an opinion and didn't really care who they offended with their words. These so-called truths contributed to the delicate state of individuals' mental health because of fear and uncertainty.

I spoke to someone who shared that a member of their community was notorious for spreading misinformation about the virus—shoving their beliefs down people's throats and condemning all forms of vaccinations, regardless of whether it is immunizations for babies, children, or the COVID-19 vaccine. The pandemic consumed every waking moment of their life, and it still does almost three years in. Members of the community tried to reason with this individual, but this person would not back down from what they believed to be the truth. People don't want the negativity or the scaremongering tactics to hold them hostage. My take on this is this: it is for freedom that you are set free. Stand firm, then, and do not let yourselves be burdened again by a yoke of slavery (Galatians 5:1).

Also, guess what? The world and your life, whether you like it or not, have forever changed because of the pandemic. Our minds have been rewired to think about our actions and how what we do or say may affect those around us. We can embrace the changes that have been implemented, or we can continue living in a bubble. Positive choices lead to opportunities to enrich not only our lives but also our overall mental and physical health and well-being. We have not been left unequipped.

> **If any lacks wisdom, let him ask of God, who gives to all liberally and without reproach, and it will be given to him. But let him ask in faith, with no doubting, for he who doubts is like a wave of the sea driven and tossed by the wind.**
>
> **James 1:5–6 (NKJV)**

Turning the Focus to Mental Health

I have touched on and hinted at the topic of emotional health since the introduction. I referred to the novelty of being restricted to your home, eventually wearing thin. Realization starts setting in that the pandemic was in no hurry to move along. It was here to stay and run its course, or at least until someone could figure out how to curb the spread. Until a barrier could be created, you were stuck at home and forced to be apart from family and friends. Stay-at-home or lock-down restrictions prevented individuals from spending time with family and friends. These restrictions also gave individuals more time to let their minds wander to dark and dreary thoughts such as the financial implications, job security, or the health of those nearest and dearest to them.

There was a dramatic surge in mental health awareness of essential workers, first-ponderers, and adult caregivers. It is challenging, on any given day, to be one of these individuals. Throw in a pandemic, separation, isolation, and endless restrictions—and you have a recipe that will have you standing to attention. On a normal, pandemic-free day everyone would go home, have a shower, enjoy a leisurely meal with the family, and get much-needed rest. The tables have been turned, and many of these individuals found themselves being separated from their families so as not to cross-contaminate those who were being cared for and to keep their families safe. It is believed that many of these people turned to substance abuse to numb their feelings. I also believe that, with the isolation and separation, there were thoughts of taking their lives or self-harming. A study showed that the rate of suspected suicides and suicide attempts by poisoning among young people rose sharply during the pandemic. A clear proof of a lack of hope for many. We do not usually learn that Christ is all we need until we reach that place where He is all we have. "Wilt thou trust him, because his strength is great? Or wilt thou leave thy labor to him? Wilt thou believe him, that he will bring home thy seed, and gather it into thy barn?" (Job 39:11–12, KJV).

Truly, our souls find rest in Him, and our salvation comes from Him. The psalmist confesses in Psalm 63:1–5 (NIV),

> **You, God, are my God, earnestly I seek you; I thirst for you, my whole being longs for you, in a dry and parched land where there is no water. I have seen you in the sanctuary and beheld your power and glory. Because your love is better than life, my lips will glorify you. I will praise you as long as I live …I will be fully satisfied as with the riches of food.**

He confidently invites all, "O taste and see that the LORD is good: blessed is the man that trusteth in him" (Psalm 34:8, KJV).

We live in a world that relies on technology to simplify our lives. Our mobile devices have apps that cater to all (or most) of our needs. We can order food or do our shopping with a swipe here and a click there and have it arrive on our doorstep. We also have an array of apps that are beneficial to our physical and mental health. These apps allow you to track your sleeping patterns, and your movement or steps. You can also track your dietary requirements, such as how much protein, fat, carbs, or water you are consuming. The Play Stores on your mobile devices have apps for absolutely anything. Find yourself an awareness app that will provide you with the necessary contact details you may need, as well as self-help tips and tricks. Utilize these tools until you can get to a medical professional to diagnose your condition, as well as suggest treatment plans that will benefit you. Glorify is an app for daily devotionals to gain strength. PrayerMate is a more traditional app that helps you register your prayer request. The Trinity Broadcasting Network and Abide are also perfect apps to help you get directions. Don't dismiss potential mental breakdown concerns as not important because I can assure you that you are important to your friends, family, and community and to God's purpose for your life.

Pandemic Heroes

We have many pandemic heroes who have played and still do play an important role during these difficult times. The media called these pandemic heroes "essential workers" or "first-ponderers" because they were dealing with infected patients. Nurses, doctors, paramedics, the clergy, and fire and rescue were the first point of contact when people suspected that they had contracted the Coronavirus. These pandemic heroes sacrificed more than anyone would ever realize. They had to work for hours on end, tending to individuals who had tested positive and were receiving medical care for severe symptoms.

These same pandemic heroes were forced to spend time away from their families, as previously mentioned, to keep everyone safe from being infected. They worked tirelessly to help care for their patients and congregations while having to stay healthy themselves. It is only a matter of time before exhaustion takes its toll. Our pandemic heroes find themselves at the rear end of a burnout or mental breakdown that has them incapable of working. This is something that can happen to anyone who throws themselves into work and neglects their mental and physical health because they have tasks to do. In humility, they considered others better than themselves, doing nothing out of selfish ambition or vain conceit nor looking not only to their own interest but also to the interests of others (Philippians 2:3–4).

Healthcare workers, as we have seen, were thrown into the deep end of the pool when the pandemic landed on their doorsteps. They experienced a new level of dedication that they hadn't been prepared for. Hospitals reached the maximum capacity of patients they could accommodate. Many countries opened temporary facilities to accommodate the overflow of COVID-19 patients, and nurses came out of retirement to help care for patients. Thankfully, after months of tracking the rise and fall of COVID-19 infections, things started settling down in the pandemic department. The headless chickens were finding their heads again.

I spoke to a healthcare worker who worked with the elderly. They had to move into the facility to be with their charges. The changes involved them going home for three days but not going anywhere or seeing anyone other than the people living in their homes. In this instance, their spouse had to quarantine for two days because they could go home. Their children, who were away at college, were not allowed in their homes during the duration of the restrictions. The healthcare worker told me that they reached a point where they felt defeated and wanted to throw in the towel. They also said that they sat staring at a bottle of vodka every evening while contemplating their future as an essential worker. This individual was always upbeat, laughing, and found the positives in everything; then, they found their mental health at an all-time low. They said that the pandemic brought out the worst in those who were isolated from their families. I asked what happened with the bottle of vodka and with plenty of laughter was told that it has a special place in the display cabinet to remind them that the solution to emotional well-being concerns does not lie in the bottom of a bottle.

Healthcare workers and religious leaders were all applauded and praised for their dedication and hard work. I believe that it is safe to say that we have a new appreciation for our pandemic heroes.

Working Remotely

One of the biggest changes to come from the pandemic was that of working remotely. Companies had to learn how to think out of the box if they wanted to keep their businesses running. Working remotely was not an option for many businesses, such as restaurants, hairdressers, or beauty salons. It was an ideal solution for the corporate world, and many embraced this change and felt a sense of relief that they still had work. However, many were concerned about the balance between working remotely and separating their family life from work. This is another one of those novelties that wore off very quickly, and employees learned that they needed to set some boundaries.

It was important to have and maintain regular office hours, as one would have when working from their place of employment. Employers had to learn to respect their employees' boundaries and stay on a schedule. Many employees struggled with the concept of "switching off" after a day of work and went over and above what was expected of them.

Imagine that your home—the place you go to after a busy day at the office—becomes your workplace. How do you separate work and home life? It is understandable and commendable that people wanted to impress their peers with their commitment to work from home, but that means setting expectations very high. Those high expectations lead to burnout for many.

The effects of the pandemic tapered down, the number of infections was significantly reduced, and slowly, the restrictions were allowing businesses and companies to start operating normally. Decisions had to be made about whether it was a feasible practice to continue working remotely. It took some adjustments, but employees found themselves preferring to work remotely, and productivity increased. Working remotely also cuts down on expenses, such as the costs involved in commuting and shopping for clothing. Businesses were also at the receiving end, where they were saving on power and office supplies. My overall impression of remote working indicated that employees were more relaxed, and after ironing out all the initial kinks at the beginning of the pandemic, boundaries were established and respected.

The first couple of months of the pandemic recorded, for example, that approximately 83 percent of Americans were working remotely (Tate, 2022). The following two years saw restrictions being lifted and many businesses returning to normal capacity. It is believed that, at the beginning of 2022, approximately 45 percent of American employees were either full- or part-time remote workers. Additional surveys indicated that approximately 91 percent of remote workers were hoping to carry on as they had been since the start of the pandemic. It is also believed that working remotely alleviates daily stress, such as commuting or distractions in the workplace. Furthermore, the surveys indicated that three out of ten remote workers would leave their positions if they were forced to physically return to their place of work. Others said that they wouldn't mind taking a cut in their salary if it meant that they could continue working from home.

I think that it is safe to say that the first year of the pandemic saw individuals struggling to balance their work and home lives. Mental health conditions spiraled as employees learned how to

Chapter 2: Exploring the Pandemic-Altered Society

navigate the obstacles they were presented with. The second year of the pandemic saw most employees happy with their working conditions, with some even opting for a permanent solution. I have met with many remote workers, and I have noticed remarkable changes in their demeanor and the way they interact with others. Let's not be fooled or made to believe that it is always sunshine and roses when working remotely. The dishes, laundry, and housecleaning still must be done—those tasks alone are enough to give anyone severe concern.

Overview of an Altered Pandemic Society

The list of changes that we have experienced since the outbreak of COVID-19 is never-ending. The world has been put through the wringer, and the population has had to adjust as best they could. Many of the changes were hard to adapt to because not everyone understood the ramifications of a pandemic. I have previously mentioned that the elderly, who are set in their ways, didn't understand why they couldn't see their families or hang out with their friends. Those in nursing homes believed that their families had given up on them because no one could visit or take them out for a stroll through the park.

I had a client who told me that their grandmother couldn't understand why no one was visiting her. They tried to communicate with the family over the phone, but that confused her even more. The nurses would report that she would sit at the front door and wait for her family to visit. Her nightmares were becoming a reality. It wasn't long before her mental health started deteriorating, and it became so bad that no one could speak to her. She was moved to another care facility during the height of the pandemic, where she peacefully passed on at the ripe old age of ninety-four.

Other changes that people struggled to understand were Zoom doctor's appointments and consultations. How can a doctor diagnose a sinus infection through a computer screen? We suddenly found ourselves in a futuristic world that resembled a science fiction movie. I'm almost sure that we can add natural disasters into the scenario, and we have a pandemic bestseller. We must break the ice and poke fun every now and again, or else we will all be permanent residents of our therapists. While I joined many in not grasping the concept of physical health telemedicine conferences, I fully supported the introduction of Zoom therapy or online church communal services. Many found these very helpful, especially for people who were struggling to cope with the isolation.

Another of my clients lived alone, and they were content with their living conditions. They would go to their local corner store once a week. Their weekly ritual abruptly stopped when their car broke down, and they didn't have the finances to afford the repair. Suddenly, their independence had been stolen from them, and they found themselves in a dark space. They started having severe anxiety attacks that were debilitating. Their heart would feel as if it was trying to break through their chest, their body ached from shaking, and they felt defeated. These attacks resulted in migraines that blinded them for up to three days at a time. Family and friends told this person to stop faking the anxiety attacks for attention. This person eventually reached out to their local emergency room and explained the situation. They were transferred to a psychiatric consultant who listened, asked questions, and eventually presented them with options. One of the options didn't sound appealing, which was taking medication; the other was the most intriguing: once-a-week Zoom therapy sessions. The therapy sessions lasted about nine months, and the consultant said that they had mastered the skill of mental self-care. Everyone needs someone to listen. Often, we are oblivious to the ready help we have (John 15:5). We can hardly live fruitful and satisfactory lives outside this truth. I have personally proven the veracity of this fact now more than ever before.

My personal takeaway from the height of the pandemic is how everyone believed that they were superior and more "educated" than those who could type just a couple of keywords into the search engines. I witnessed nastiness among people who forced their beliefs and opinions on others. The biggest drama—even bigger than soap operas give us—was surrounding the vaccine. Everyone jumped on some kind of bandwagon to share their views. I witnessed friendships being threatened and harmful words being flung around. I had to insert a filter in front of my mouth to keep myself in check. I don't like confrontations, and I certainly don't like it when I see people being attacked for having an opinion that varies from someone else. No one is going to force you to do something you don't want to do, but no one else has the right to be a bully about the choices someone else makes. People need to remember that harmful words and actions can never be retracted. Once they leave your mouth and land in someone's ear, it is too late to take it back. You can spend a lifetime saying sorry, but those words will always be hanging around. We should never forget the saying, "The soothing tongue is a tree of life, but a perverse tongue crushes the spirit" (Proverbs 15:4, NIV).

The End of the Pandemic

Do we go planning any post-pandemic parties just yet? It may feel as if the pandemic is over, especially if you ignore the mainstream media, but there is no total light at the end of any tunnels right now. The first two years of the pandemic saw various strains of the COVID-19 virus cause spikes in the number of infections. It appears COVID-19 had a vendetta it wanted to settle each time the restrictions were eased. Many countries found themselves on a seesaw, where the restrictions were eased and tightened so many times that people ended up putting themselves into lockdown.

The introduction of the vaccine—love it or hate it—may have helped with slowing down the number of infections. It is important to note that the vaccine is not a cure for the COVID-19 virus. The vaccine was not created to prevent the virus; it was meant to build up immune systems. I have seen many people say that they can't get measles, mumps, or chickenpox because they have been vaccinated as children. I also have met adults in their thirties who have had mumps, measles, and chicken pox—and the backlash they receive from people who think they know everything is overwhelming to anyone. You feel as if you are being personally attacked when people tell you that you are false.

We stepped into a whole new world at the end of 2019. The world that we knew was changing at the rate of a wildfire. The new world, although it looked the same, was unfamiliar as we had to learn how to apply the changes that were handed down to us. The first couple of weeks were like a vacation, and everyone was baking banana and sourdough bread. Talk show hosts were presenting their shows from the comfort of their homes and connecting with their co-hosts via satellite connections. Our new world has evolved with its many changes and transformations.

"When will the pandemic be over?" This is a question that doesn't have an answer in our new world. No one can give a definitive answer. We live in faith, hope, and belief that the pandemic will eventually fizzle out forever. We must let the pandemic run its course. Hopefully, in the not-too-distant future, the CDC and

Chapter 2: Exploring the Pandemic-Altered Society

WHO will announce that no new variants of the Coronavirus exist and that there have been no new infections for more than thirty days. We all must hold fast to the profession of our faith without wavering, regardless of the circumstances or what we think we see or experience (Hebrews 10:23). Difficult times can leave us feeling exposed and unprotected. However, God offers us security that isn't dependent on our situation. "Those who know your name trust in you, for you, LORD, have never forsaken those who seek you" (Psalm 9:10, NIV). We can trust Him to sustain us, provide for us, and be with us even amid our hardships. There will be hard times (John 16:33), but He will always be with you (Matthew 28:20). This is the profession of our faith.

CHAPTER 3:

Exploring the Struggles of Adjusting to the Whole New World

"Be very careful, then, how you live—not as unwise but as wise, making the most of every opportunity"

(Ephesians 5:15–16, NIV).

"In the midst of chaos, there is also opportunity"

(Sun Tzu).

There is no denying that the world was thrust into bubbles when news of the pandemic was released at the end of 2019. Scientists, researchers, immunologists, and a whole team of medical professionals got together to work on a solution to slow the spread and build up immunities. Many renewed their strength day by day in the knowledge that those who trust in the Lord shall renew their strength like an eagle. They will run and not grow weary; they will walk and not faint (Isaiah 40:31). Government officials did what they could under the direction of WHO, the CDC, and local health organizations across the globe. Mandates were issued, and temporary laws were put into place to ensure that citizens knew that if lines were crossed, there would be repercussions. People felt intimidated and overwhelmed by the changes, and many referred to the restrictions as being draconian laws. A quick look at my trusted online dictionary, Merriam-Webster, tells us that "draconian" is defined as cruel or severe. The definition most definitely adds fuel to the fire of how people were feeling about the restrictions and mandates (Merriam-Webster).

I previously mentioned some of the "laws" that were put into place and enforced on millions of people. The purchase of cigarettes or any form of nicotine products was prohibited for approximately five months. This was done to get people to stop smoking and to keep them away from the shops. The ban backfired on the government because it opened a secret door to the black-market trading of tobacco products, which cost the government millions in revenue and taxes. The same fate was imposed on the sale of alcohol, which lasted a little longer than the tobacco ban, and on congregational assemblies. Other restrictions included walking or playing on the beach, and curfews were put in place. We can see why many people referred to the restrictions and temporary laws as being draconian.

Chapter 3: Exploring the Struggles of Adjusting to the Whole New World

A year into the pandemic saw restrictions being eased ever so slightly. The world found itself on a roller coaster during the surges and drops of infections. New variants of the virus were discovered, and the reins were tightened until a noticeable decrease in infections was detected. Many countries lifted the mandate of wearing face masks, but others were still firmly in place. Inching towards the second year of the pandemic, people were allowed to resume congregational meetings except with conditions such as wearing face masks, retaining the six-foot distance apart, and adhering to the limit for indoor gatherings.

It wasn't too long after these changes that just about all restrictions and mandates were lifted. I had someone tell me that they felt as if people didn't care that the risk of the Coronavirus was still alive and thriving. They proceeded to tell me that they had suffered through four bouts of the virus in two years. My editor and her family have just been through their second bout of the virus, and it hit them hard. This makes me reflect on the meaning of life and what our future looks like. But what does the Lord desire and plan for us?

> **"For I know the plans I have for you," declares the LORD, "plans to prosper you and not to harm you, plans to give you hope and a future. Then you will call on me and come and pray to me, and I will listen to you. You will seek me and find me when you seek me with all your heart."**
>
> **Jeremiah 29:11–13 (NIV)**

This is very uplifting.

The Meaning of Life—Through the Eyes of Pandemic Warriors

You, me, and everyone throughout the world are pandemic warriors. We walked the walk and talked the talk, and we got to share our experiences—good or bad—with future generations. It was up to us to educate our children and ourselves on how to adapt to this new world we found ourselves in. The pandemic presented us with the perfect opportunity to reassess the direction in which our lives were going. The other side of the pandemic coin saw people feeling as if they no longer had any purpose in life. I found that many people were angry about the situations they were in.

I do understand that people were and are still angry. We must ask the question: Who are we angry with? This question leads us to play the "blame game," where the buck is passed around, and no one takes responsibility. I believe that no one person, country, or government organization is responsible for the pandemic. It is one of those natural disasters, as previously mentioned, that happens without prior notice. Everyone was in uncharted waters as they were trying to figure out an escape plan to navigate through the obstacles that COVID-19 brought with it.

It took a while for those in charge to create a plan that "worked" for each country. There were many hits and misses along the way, but somehow—no matter how reluctant we were—we earned the title of pandemic warriors. Many complied with and respected the restrictions imposed; especially if it meant keeping our high-risk families safe from infection. Others were a little less reluctant to comply, but they found ways to interact with their loved ones without putting them at risk. Then, we have those who defied and disrespected the restrictions because they didn't believe that COVID-19 and all the statistics were truthful. I'm not here to choose sides or point fingers. I have said multiple

Chapter 3: Exploring the Struggles of Adjusting to the Whole New World

times that everyone has the freedom of choice, and no one can force you to believe in something you don't want to. I'm here to understand how the pandemic affected people, made them think about life, and how everyone coped with the changes in their life situations.

Exploring the Meaning of Life in a Pandemic World

In November 2021, researchers, assistants, and analysts from the Pews Research Center created public surveys to understand how the population felt about the pandemic (Silver et al., 2021). This was when restrictions were being eased, and people could resume the new normal lives they had become accustomed to. One of the questions featured in the survey was about the pandemic life and what people were experiencing. They also wanted to know how and where individuals found meaning in the new life that had turned their worlds upside down. Everyone had an opinion—with some being positive, others not, and the fence-sitters. We must remember that it is impossible to please everyone, and there will always be those who choose to live in "Doom-and-Gloomville" and those who opt to thrive and prosper in "Happyville."

Individuals from "Happyville" believed that the pandemic gave them an excellent opportunity to reflect on how they had been living their lives. These are people who pushed themselves to the limit at work—those who had households that relied on getting everyone up and ready for school, taking children to school, running around to extramural activities, and still making sure everyone was fed, had clean clothes, and a tidy house. Many said that they welcomed the stay-at-home or lock-down orders because they allowed them to operate at a slower pace. Others said that they had time to reflect and take stock of their lives and make some much-needed changes that would benefit everyone involved. The biggest takeaway from "Happyville" was that people learned to appreciate their lives; partners could see what it took to keep everything running like a well-oiled machine, and children could appreciate the effort their parents and caregivers went through to provide them with everything they needed or wanted.

I want to introduce you to "Helperville." This quaint but loving community is where individuals become united. Everyone comes together to help someone in need. One of the respondents of the survey was from Taiwan, and they said, like every Christian community, that their community was always ready and willing to help during a crisis such as the pandemic, earthquakes, or landslides. I like to think that "Helperville" exists in all communities. I have spoken to many people who have been in a position where they didn't have money to put food on the table, and communities stepped up and donated whatever they could. The individual from Taiwan hit the ball out of the park when they said that everyone stands together to help those in need. Welcome to the community of "Helperville," which spreads anonymous cheer to those who require assistance.

Then, we have our community members from "Doom-and-Gloomville," who don't seem to see any positive meaning in their lives. They will complain that they can't go anywhere or do anything and that they are prisoners in their homes. They have expressed that nothing satisfies them because their freedom has been taken away from them. I suspect that this is a community that spends time following conspiracy theory websites and buys into the negativity being spread. These are also the people I want to reach out to and address their challenges because they are struggling to cope with the changes of the new world. I know that "Doom-and-Gloomville" has been a safe haven for many, especially for those who struggle because of the lives of family or friends taken by the pandemic.

Remember, our hope or strength is not in man but in the power of the promises and reassurances of God. Our comfort in our pains is in His promises to preserve us. He is near to those who are discouraged; He saves those who have lost all hope (Psalm 34:18). He is with us when we are crushed in spirit; He will strengthen us, help us, and uphold us and will not forsake us (Isaiah 41:10). Our confidence and hope should grow in the power of His words and promises that He is with us, loving us, walking alongside us amid our sorrows, and nothing can separate us from His love (Romans 8:31–39), not even the pain of bereavement. So no, there will be no judgment from me or anybody against you. But I do hope that one day, you will find your way to "Happyville" and "Helperville." You will be welcomed with open, loving, and caring arms.

Facing Challenges During the Search for the Meaning of Life

It is difficult to be positive when it feels as if you are being used as target practice by the world. Social media influencers portray a world where everything is perfect, and nothing is out of place on their immaculate hair extensions and false eyelashes. I scrolled through some family vlogs on YouTube to see and understand if these "perfect" people face any challenges; the best I could come up with were some nails being broken or tomato stains on stone tiles. I think it is safe to say that life, in general, is not all about chocolate-covered strawberries and champagne. Whoever told us that, by the way? The real world has real challenges, and this is where it becomes difficult to find a positive response to the meaning of life outside the grace provided by the power of God.

You are going to have your eternal optimists, who will constantly tell you that everything is going to be fine or that everything will work out the way it should. Yes, those are a couple of phrases we have all heard one too many times, and I understand that this is not something you want to hear; many of us can't help but have hope that everything will be good again. I am a core optimist and believer; I rely on and believe strongly in the power of God's promises. I believe I can do all things through Him who gives me strength (Philippians 4:13), and He who guides and makes my life pleasant and my future bright (Psalm 16:6). I believe that everything is going to be fine, and this strong faith has always worked for me.

I recently spoke to someone who was retrenched from their job at the start of the pandemic. Everyone around them was falling apart, but they remained hopeful and positive, and a month later, they found what they believed to be their dream job. They started feeling the pressure of the economy and knew that they needed to find something to supplement their income. They manifested their desire to find another job in the middle of 2022, and at the beginning of 2023, they were approached by the company that retrenched them. They were invited to join the company, along with one other individual who was retrenched. You can remain strong, knowing that even if things look gloomy now, be rest assured that God has plans for you, a future filled with hope.

Challenges that individuals were plagued with were job losses, financial hardships, the breakdown of personal relationships or marriages, and concerns about the health and well-being of loved ones. These are challenges that are happening in the real world and are a reminder that what we see on social media may not be real. The real world is where people are fighting for survival; they worry about their finances and whether they will have enough

Chapter 3: Exploring the Struggles of Adjusting to the Whole New World

money to pay the bills. The real world is not as some make it out to be, but it is the most beautiful place in your world when you are looking for the silver lining around the darkest clouds. Find your meaning in life by adopting positivity amongst the challenges (Silver et al., 2021).

Find Your Meaning of Life

Don't give society permission to dictate how you should be living your life. It is not our fault that we found ourselves in a global pandemic. We have choices, and we can choose to be angry at everyone and everything because the pandemic had the audacity to settle down in our town. We have had to learn a lot over the last couple of COVID-19 years. Education and work were a whole new experience where we had to rely on Zoom, Microsoft Teams, or Skype to communicate with teachers, bosses, and co-workers. Talk show hosts, such as Ellen DeGeneres and Jimmy Kimmel, worked via satellite to stream their content to viewers. The show had to go on; children had to be educated or face repeating another year in their grade, and employers needed to keep their companies from going under.

I can't tell you what your meaning in life should be. That is something you must figure out for yourself. Make some lists with goals that you would like to accomplish. Pick ones that speak to your heart and soul. The pandemic taught me that life is precious and far too fragile. We take so much for granted that we don't stop to think about the important fragments that make up our lives. We expect our family members and friends to live forever, but the truth is that no one does. Make peace with those who hurt your feelings, apologize to those you may have offended, and show everyone kindness.

One of my clients told me that they found a renewed meaning in life when a family member passed on after having a stroke. They were very close, which resulted in my client retreating into a dark, hard shell. Their anxiety attacks returned with a vengeance. They found themselves stuck between extreme anger and sadness. They were not interested in looking for the light at the end of the tunnel. It is ironic to note that they found their meaning in life through pain. This is not the type of pain you experience when cutting or burning yourself; it is the pain of being betrayed and lied to. The discovery of what family members were doing and saying is what kicked my client out of the dark, hard shell. They knew that their relationship with their deceased family member meant more than wallowing in the destruction of their life. They needed not to grieve as those who do not have hope. We are taught not to be ignorant concerning those who have fallen asleep, lest we sorrow as others who have no hope. "For if we believe that Jesus died and rose again, even so God will bring with Him those who sleep in Jesus" (1 Thessalonians 4:14, NKJV).

Your meaning in life can be anything that makes you feel valued. Look into the mirror and know that the person looking back at you is your meaning in life. You need to look after that person, and when you have mastered the art of loving and respecting, you can move on to goals to find your next meaning in life. Let's give the pandemic a little bit of praise—not too much—but enough to thank it for allowing us to slow down and appreciate the life we have. Love it or hate it, the pandemic taught us some valuable lessons and presented us with way too many challenges, but we weathered the storm, and we will continue tailgating whatever pandemic storms may follow.

CHAPTER 4:

Utilizing the Voice of Reason to Embrace Changes

"Remember ye not the former things, neither consider the things of old"

(Isaiah 43:18, KJV).

"Change is the law of life. And those who look only to the past or present are certain to miss the future"

(John F. Kennedy).

Changes are overwhelming and intimidating, especially when we are forced out of our comfort zone. I introduced you to the fear of change in chapter 1. I highlighted the difficulties many people face when the mention of change is uttered. We try to resist, but at the end of a very long battle, we realize that we either must adapt or fall behind. I will be the first to admit that changes are scary and that I am not the only one in this position of uncertainty. Realization becomes the voice of reason when I notice that I am not the only one bobbing up and down on a life raft to avoid making changes.

Changes are scary, but we all have a choice about how they will affect us. We can live in fear as the necessary changes are implemented around us without our consent, or we can let go of the life raft, swim to the shore, and hit the ground running. Changes will affect everyone differently, and it is a matter of taking stock of the situations you are presented with. This chapter is about coping and adjusting to the changes you were forced to adopt when news of the pandemic surfaces. I have previously mentioned that we were approaching uncharted waters, and we had to learn to cope with the myriad of changes. It is no secret that many of us struggled at the start of the pandemic, and slowly but surely, we found our groove and worked on ways to build our resilience.

The quote at the beginning of the chapter spoke to my soul. My interpretation of it is that if you don't make the necessary changes to enrich your life, you can't move past the barrier that takes you to the next phase of your life. The take is I must be transformed by the renewing of my mind. Sometimes, the scariest changes can lead to the greatest growth in our lives. I have found myself on the receiving end of narcissistic relationships and have been dealing with friends and family who have bipolar disorder. What message am I sending to my family, friends, and readers if I don't simplify my life by accepting and making peace with changes? I'm not going to allow the pandemic to hold me hostage against my will, and I am most definitely not going to let fear hold me back. I am an advocate for positivity, and I am more than willing to lead us through our fear of change. Even as we learn to cope with changes, become resilient, and embrace the fear of normality.

Implementing Tools to Cope with Change

The beginning of the pandemic saw an increase in emotional health concerns such as depression, panic, and anxiety. The beginning was full of uncertainty, and I believe that many adjusted to the rules and regulations. We may not have been jumping for joy about all the restrictions and changes, but nonetheless, we made sweet lemonade with the lemons that were thrown at us. I have experienced that a lot of people were focused on how their lives would be affected during the stay-at-home orders or lockdown restrictions. It was as if no one stopped to think and expand their views to the possibility that all the mandates and restrictions would eventually be eased and phased to blend in without the protection of their bubbles. I'm not talking about the ending of the pandemic, but I am referring to easing into a new normal.

I spoke to individuals who were not very confident about adjusting to the new normal. One person even told me that it took them two years to get used to the idea of having the upper hand in denying people from entering their property or their homes. They had adapted to the pandemic rules and regulations and discovered that they preferred not having visitors stop by whenever they wanted. They said that whenever the restrictions were being eased, they felt their anxiety growing. The day finally arrived when all government restrictions and mandates had fallen away; international travel borders were reopened, public gatherings were permitted, in-school education was resumed, and individuals could return to their places of work. The individual told me that their anxiety levels exceeded their early day pandemic levels because the fear of resuming a "normal" life was even more overwhelming than being restricted to their home.

Why would you be more anxious when given more freedom?

What is holding you back from finding your ray of sunshine in the whole new world?

What would you do to make yourself feel comfortable with your newfound freedom?

The answers to these questions are going to help you design a pathway that is tailor-made for you. It is going to help you cope without the protection from the bubble world you have found comfort in. The time has arrived to give you some handy-dandy tools to carve your pedestal that will tell the world that you won't be a hostage in your whole new world. Are you ready to embrace the changes?

Breaking the Fear of Normal Barriers

The fear of normal carries a little more weight than anyone realizes. You may have accepted that restrictions and mandates have fallen away. This is something that everyone—regardless of demographics—has experienced, and many have embraced. We are slowly getting used to going to the store without wearing a face mask. It is lovely to see people's smiles and grumpy disapproval glares. We have all this freedom handed to us on silver platters, yet we are apprehensive. One would imagine that anxiety, depression, and concern would have eased along with

Chapter 4: Utilizing the Voice of Reason to Embrace Changes

the restrictions, but sadly, this is not the case. The truth is that people are afraid to let down their defenses because mainstream media reports on new variants of the Coronavirus, new infections, hospitalizations, and deaths.

I remember how I felt the first time I went to Target without my face mask. My heart was trying to escape through my throat. Beads of sweat emerged from every pore on my body to form tidal pools. The feeling of guilt was real. I utilized one of my coping techniques to slow my breathing and allow my heart to settle down. I had to break down the barrier of guilt and realize that I wasn't defying any orders. I was given permission to retire my face mask—knowing that I wouldn't be pelted with stones for not following a protocol that was drummed into us since the beginning of 2022. It is easy to understand why many people are having a hard time accepting the new normal and why they are afraid—many countries threatened their citizens with fines or jail time if they didn't comply with the regulations.

Erring on the Side of Worry

I like to think that we are a nation of problem-solvers. We want to be the hero who steps up to the plate to make life as easy as possible. We even go so far as to carry the world and its problems on our shoulders. Many of us believe that we must be like Atlas when, in reality, we are expected to be who we are—normal, (semi) well-adjusted human beings.

I would, once more, like to refer to the quote at the beginning of the chapter, which says that we need to stop living in the past. Did you know—this may come as a shock to many—that you cannot go back to the past to change what has happened? I know this comes as a massive surprise and shock to you, but that is the reality of the life we find ourselves in. We cannot change the past because it has happened, and the t-shirt was worn, burned, and buried at that stage of our lives. Forget those things that are behind, and reach out to those good things to come, lest you miss the new things yet to come. "Forget the former things; do not dwell on the past. See, I am doing a new thing! Now it springs up; do you not perceive it?" (Isaiah 43:18–19, NIV).

The beginning of the pandemic also brought a lot of "what ifs" that were sparked by comments from government health officials. The uncertainty that we were faced with was met with "what ifs," which had people questioning not only their health but that of their families and friends. We saw that healthcare and essential workers were in the line of fire, and many had to be isolated from their families so that they didn't jeopardize the health and well-being of their loved ones, colleagues, patients, or themselves. The worry barrier goes a little further than being concerned about health; it includes the stress of worrying about where the next meal will come from, gang and gun violence, and political agendas. I want to implore you to be present in your life. Adopt a new outlook on life that promotes positiveness during the dark and dreary times we are experiencing. The world may have changed, but it is a continuous cycle that increases your anxiety and stress levels. I want you to know that you don't have to be the hero all the time. Worry is like a rocking chair. It keeps you going, but you don't get anywhere.

"Take therefore no thought for the morrow: for the morrow shall take thoughts for the things of itself. Sufficient unto the day is the evil thereof" (Matthew 6:34, KJV).

"If God so clothe the grass of the field, which to day is, and to morrow is cast into the oven, shall he not much more clothe you?" (Matthew 6:30, KJV).

Chapter 4: Utilizing the Voice of Reason to Embrace Changes

Introducing Positivity

I have previously mentioned that I am an eternal optimist who sees the good in everything. This, more than anything, has to do with my strong and proven faith in the power of God and in His possibilities. I have tested and proven it. I also believe that there is a time and place for everything. To everything under the heavens, there is a season, and a time to every purpose.

> **A time to be born, and a time to die; a time to plant, and a time to pluck up that which is planted; A time to kill, and a time to heal; a time to break down, and a time to build up; A time to weep, and a time to laugh; a time to mourn, and a time to dance; A time to cast away stones, and a time to gather stones together; a time to embrace, and a time to refrain from embracing; A time to get, and a time to lose; a time to keep, and a time to cast away; A time to rend, and a time to sew; a time to keep silence, and a time to speak; A time to love, and a time to hate; a time of war, and a time of peace.**
>
> **Ecclesiastes 3:2–8 (KJV)**

This is very instructive for our psychological and emotional well-being. Now is the time in our lives to bounce back after the adversity that tailed the pandemic. Now is the time to renew our strength like that of an eagle and transit into the new post-pandemic era with resilience, a transformed mindset, and judgment. This strengthens my positive energy. I'm not going to be unreasonable and force my beliefs on you. I know what it is like to have no faith in humanity and not trust what is being shared. I have been there before, and I have multiple t-shirts that have been burned and buried.

One of the most important lessons to learn is that we can't stop the inevitable from happening. I don't buy into conspiracy theories because then I would be feeding my anxiety, and I would be stuck in the black hole of fear for the rest of my life. I want to help you break free from the clutches of anxiety. The only way to address your worries and conquer your fears is to change the way you think about what works for you. Slow and steady will get you to the finish line, but I want you to know that this is not a race. I would like to share some helpful tips that will assist in introducing confidence and positivity into your life:

Treat yourself with the respect you deserve. Love yourself and extend the love to your neighbors (Matthew 22:39). Treat yourself with kindness, compassion, and respect. Knowing that Christ already sees you as the perfect reflection of Himself (1 John 3:1–3).

Be mindful of your needs to be happy. Knowing that true gladness comes from the presence of God (Acts 2:28).

Get some rest. Your mind, body, and soul need sufficient rest so that it may be refreshed. Always return to your rest (Exodus 23:12). It is easy to get swept up, forgetting the importance of taking a moment to give time to renewal (Psalm 116:7).

Practice yoga or invest a couple of dollars for an online exercise module. Training your body is of value, promising benefits in this life and in the life to come (1 Timothy 4:8).

Meditate when you are feeling overwhelmed. Meditate on whatever things are true, whatever things are noble, whatever things are just, whatever things are pure, whatever things are lovely, whatever things are of good report, if there is any virtue and if

Chapter 4: Utilizing the Voice of Reason to Embrace Changes

there is anything praiseworthy—meditate on these things, just as we are taught in Philippians 4:8.

Practice breathing techniques to ease your anxiety levels. Do not be anxious about anything (Philippians 4:6).

Practice daily positive affirmations, build up your self-esteem, and avoid self-sabotage (Psalm 141:3).

Adopt a self-care routine that will make you feel special.

Last, but not the least, have a conversation with the person looking back at you from the mirror. Examine and rejoice in yourself (Galatians 6:3–4). Self-reflection not only helps us integrate into our daily lives but allows us to look for God in our lives.

Learning How to Cope with Change

We have determined that implementing changes is not as easily accepted as some may believe. It is harder for the older generation to make changes on a whim because they have created comfortable lives for themselves. The onset and invasion of the pandemic had rules that had to be implemented without much notice. I spoke to a lady who told me that she was relieved that her parents had passed on several years before the pandemic. She said that her parents would not have been able to cope with the changes and, most especially, would have landed themselves in trouble for breaking all the rules. They were both very sociable people, and social distancing would not have worked in their favor. I have spoken to many people who felt the same way as this lady did, but at the end of the day, I believe that our older generation may have surprised us by adapting to their new normal.

I am dedicating this section of the chapter to those individuals who feel overwhelmed, intimidated, and like a fish out of water.

This chapter speaks into the hearts and souls of those who experience cold sweats at the mere suggestion of changing something that has been part of their lives since conception—okay, not really, but close enough. We know that changes are either received very well or met with resistance. No two individuals will have the same experience, and it would not be fair to compare people's reactions. I was never any good with change until I was helped; therefore, my heart greatly rejoiced. I built a fortress around myself and my children to protect us from any pain and suffering that may occur. It became a habit that was very difficult to veer away from as my children got older. I had to be the parent who released their children from the fortress, and no matter how hard it was to make those changes, they needed to happen.

The COVID-19 pandemic arrived with a flair for theatrics, creating panic and mass pandemonium as people rushed to the stores to stock up on toilet paper, flour, or rice. I remember watching news reports of people physically fighting to ensure they got the items they "wanted." This was the chaos that occurred around the world. Almost three years down the line, the shelves in the stores are fully stocked and no one is fighting to get toilet paper—that must have been the most bizarre pandemic "must-have" item to physically attack someone for. The fear of change doesn't take any hostages, and it can invade your comfort zone in the blink of an eye. The habits you created for yourself were crumbled into a little ball and discarded as if they never existed.

I was recently asked to identify the way I choose to cope with changes. This made me think, analyze, and create lists to help me on this quest. I would have to prepare myself mentally for any changes and do the slow-and-steady waltz before I fully implemented the Viennese waltz. The person who asked me the question explained that they had learned about two types of cop-

Chapter 4: Utilizing the Voice of Reason to Embrace Changes

ing: escape and control; evidently, I am a control coper. On one side of the fence, you have people who don't want to deal with or ignore changes that are beneficial to their lives; on the other side of the fence, you have those who want to embrace changes but need the time and support to get to where they need to be.

The Stages of Change

The loss of a loved one because of cancer, a stroke, a heart attack, or a motor vehicle accident plunges you into a very dark place. That dark place is called grief. Grief comes with various stages that will attempt to help you get through the darkest time of your life. The stages of grief will guide you toward the light as you work through your pain. I would like to share a list of the seven stages of grief that you will wade through to find the light of healing:

Not believing your new reality without your loved one, plagued by guilt that you could have said or done more for your loved one; being angry all the time, asking questions, and doing whatever you can to have your loved one back wanting to be left alone; showing no interest in self-care stepping out of the shadows; reconnecting with society healing and reconstruction as you realize that your loved one wouldn't want you to pine; the realization and acceptance that life does go on, and knowing that it is perfectly normal to laugh and be happy again because of the hope of resurrection and victory over death through Jesus Christ (1 Corinthians 15:51–56).

I shared the stages of grief to show you that your struggles with change closely mimic those of someone who is grieving. Your perfectly curated habits have been blown apart by a pandemic that has no respect for anyone. The changes you were forced to accept were traumatic. You may have felt as if the ground had opened beneath you because you didn't have time to prepare for the changes. Guess what? You may already know this little secret—you weathered the storm, and if you are reading this, then you know that it is not a very well-kept secret.

I have a friend who isn't shy and doesn't hesitate to tell me to put on my big people's underwear, tie my bootlaces, and take control of my feelings and emotions. Let's look at the typical reactions you may expect when faced with change:

> **You are in a state of shock and feel as if your head is going to spin off your shoulders.**
>
> **You are angry at the instigator of the change: in this case, COVID-19.**
>
> **You realize that you need to make peace with the changes.**
>
> **You give in and accept that change is part of your whole new world.**

You Are Stronger than You Think

Did you know that you can do anything you set your mind to? This was something I struggled to grasp when I was growing up. My family and educators would tell me that I needed to apply this, that, and the other to my skill set to prosper in the future. Everyone saw something in me that I never realized until I went to college and then transitioned to adulthood. I realized that I could do hard things, and I didn't have to rely on others to carry me—I was resilient. We can all prevail if we choose to.

I didn't back down from challenges because I was told, at a young age, that I could do anything. I didn't see myself as a superhero or Atlas, who carried the world on his shoulders, but I was doing what I needed to do to survive. I had to stand up for myself and defeat the bullies who tried to control my life.

Chapter 4: Utilizing the Voice of Reason to Embrace Changes

I am committed to doing whatever needs to be done. I committed my life to ensuring that I would care for my child the day I joined the worldwide motherhood club. I am fiercely protective and committed to my family and friends—even those who don't acknowledge me. I don't say one thing and mean something else because that goes against the code of resilience.

Are you ready to accept a challenge that will strengthen your resilience?

Are you ready to move past whatever fear is holding you hostage?

Don't give the pandemic permission to stand in the way of your strengths. It is okay to live your life safely—it is encouraged. If you suspect that you or someone you may have interacted with has been infected, take the necessary precautions without condemnation. Be patient, kind, caring, and understanding of what is going on around you. Be an example of strength and resilience because I can assure you that other people are going to need your God-given strength to help them step out and move forward.

We have reached the part of the chapter where we must take a giant leap into the next part of our journey. A new and exciting adventure is beckoning us. We will be exploring the topic of working and work conditions in our whole new world. It is safe to say that everyone experienced major upheavals during the pandemic. The world slowly got its toes wet as people re-entered the workplace, and changes were put into effect that needed to be tested by employees and employers. I'll see you in the next chapter.

CHAPTER 5:

Adjusting to Your New Workplace in the Pandemic-Altered World

"Times of transition are strenuous, but I love them. They are an opportunity to purge, rethink priorities and be intentional about new habits. We can make our new normal any way we want"

(Kristin Armstrong).

It never dawned on me that the pandemic would have an indefinite lifespan. I joined the masses by believing that the Coronavirus would be like the bird or swine flu. A couple of weeks, maybe two months at the most, and it would be contained; life would go on. The pandemic-imposed vacation was fun and exciting at the beginning, but the honeymoon phase wore off when the realization hit home that COVID-19 was serious. This virus meant business, and it didn't care who felt the effects. Employers had to think outside of many boxes to come up with a solution, ways to maintain productivity, and ensure that employees had an income.

Working remotely is not a new concept that someone came up with at the beginning of the pandemic. It has been around for many years, as far back as 1983 with a small group of IBM workers who wanted to research the effectiveness of working remotely (Butler, n.d.). I had to go searching through the dusty archives and discovered that the concept of working remotely originated as far back as 1973 by Jack Nilles, a NASA engineer. Nilles was the genius who planted a seed that would lead to opportunities that would allow billions of people to work from anywhere in the world. The term used by Nilles was "telecommuting," and I am left wondering if he ever believed that his prediction of working remotely would offer job security for billions of people during a global pandemic. Telecommuting offered more than job security; it created and provided remote work opportunities for individuals who needed to have flexible work schedules. Jack Nilles planted the seed, and fifty years later, he has made people grateful for an income in a time when the future is uncertain.

The arrival of COVID-19 opened many doors, but it also shut and sealed many others. This chapter is dedicated to adjusting to the new working conditions and dynamics that you have been introduced to. I have spoken about and referred to the struggles everyone has experienced (and still does) with the sudden changes they were introduced to. It may not be easy to adapt to something at the drop of a hat, but it is not impossible. If you look at the word impossible—what do you see? The first two letters are "im," followed by "possible," which translates to "I'm possible," which should put a huge smile on your face because it is just one of many reaffirmations to let you know that you can do all things if you believe and put your mind into it. You've weathered some scary storms since the start of the pandemic, and you keep on going.

Working from Home

I have discussed the concept of working from home in previous chapters and given you a glimpse into the origin of telecommuting. I know and have spoken to many people who have been working remotely for more than twenty years and who have said that they would never be able to work in an office. The evolution of technology has allowed for the creation of jobs in a world where people are struggling to find work outside in the real world. Desperate times call for desperate measures, especially at a time when we are living in financial hardships and the economy is struggling to regain its composure since the outbreak of COVID-19. I remember a friend telling me that they would rather work for peanuts than not be productive. They needed to keep busy or else risk the chance of ending up in that dark hole of depression I have referred to. It is important to put in effort and hard work to earn a living. "In all labor there is profit, But idle chatter leads only to poverty" (Proverbs 14:23, NKJV). A wise man knows the value of hard work and of thriftiness (Proverbs 6:6–8). It is important for our mental health to stay busy so that we don't have time to think: What if? Or how am I? You are defined by your work.

I also know and understand that many people need human interaction. Extroverts need to be in the company of others to keep their minds active. They feed off the hustle and bustle of their coworkers. And then, COVID-19 arrived, unpacked its bags, and moved in for its open-ended vacation. The arrival of this uninvited guest caused mayhem and pandemonium in all the corners of the world. Mindsets had to be changed as employers started rolling out their plans for working remotely. Everyone was keenly aware that they needed to work, but it was difficult for extroverts who needed their coworkers to spur them on and keep them motivated. It is understandable that these individuals believed that working from home was like a prison sentence.

Everyone had to learn to adjust to the new workplace dynamics. I know that many may not have jumped for joy when they were introduced to the idea of working from home for the unforeseeable future. I have heard stories of people who tried to bargain with government officials to allow them to work in their workplace if they promised to take all the necessary precautions to stay and keep others safe. The bargaining got them nowhere, and they were given two choices: either work from home or resign. I believe that this is the stage when they realized the severity of the pandemic and that they had to make the changes.

Making Sweet Lemonade Out of Sour Lemons

This was just one of those situations where we must shape up or ship out. We may not want to work from home, but we must realize that we have people who depend on our incomes. We can't throw in the towel because we don't want anything to do with the imposed changes. I have seen instances where people

Chapter 5: Adjusting to Your New Workplace in the Pandemic-Altered World

believed that if they stood up to the changes and protested, they would be the victors, and everyone would be grateful. Can I tell you a secret? Come a little closer, but be careful that you don't squint: No one, in any job, is irreplaceable. There are people who believe that no one can do their job as well as they can, but allow me to be the one to pop their flimsy bubbles and give their egos the reality check it requires—the next person will learn their jobs and might be better than their predecessors. Everyone can be replaced in the workplace, so it is a matter of accepting your new normal.

You have decided that working from home is something you need to accept if you want to keep your job. All you must do is make a couple of changes that will set you up for success. You are going to set up boundaries that are essential to a successful working-from-home environment. Your family must realize that changes are going to be essential to a happy home. The same way of thinking will apply to someone who lives alone. You need to learn how to separate your work and home life to maximize productivity and maintain positiveness. Let's look at some helpful tips to create a healthy working-from-home work environment.

Scheduling

You would have a calendar that would have your day scheduled until the day ends if you were working away from home. The same consideration will take effect when working remotely. Changes must be made that include everyone living within the confines of your home; this includes your spouse, partner, children, and non-human children. We saw the closure of schools, and many children were given the opportunity to continue their education from home. Mom and Dad had to learn to become both teachers and parents at the same time. I know of many educators who gave parents helpful information to ensure that everyone concerned was disciplined to do the tasks they were given. This is what your work-from-home needs: discipline.

You need to ensure that everyone knows what your schedule looks like. Make a million lists and put them up for everyone to see. Coordinate your schedules with everyone in your home and be considerate of any unplanned changes that may occur. I like the idea of being courteous towards your employers or supervisors and letting them know what the schedule looks like so that they, too, can know what is going on. This will make it easier for them to schedule digital face-to-face meetings via Zoom, Skype, or Microsoft Teams. You have planned your schedules, ironed out the kinks, and made the necessary provisions for unplanned changes; it is now time to figure out a good place where you can work.

Appropriate Workspace

Designate a space in your home where you can set up your workspace. Your couch and bed are not an office, and it will most definitely reflect poorly on your productivity. I had someone tell me that you need to enforce boundaries or face the risk of burnout, especially if you are new to working from home. That is something that many people struggled with at the beginning of the pandemic when they were informed that they would be working from home. Creating a workspace and having boundaries are important for your mental health and productivity. Keep your office out of your bedroom to avoid the temptation to crawl under the covers on a chilly winter's day.

You can cordon off a corner in your lounge or even the kitchen, where you can put a small desk and have all your office supplies on hand. I would suggest that all remote workers invest in noise-canceling headphones to block out distractions. Ensure that you have everything you need within your reach to minimize having to jump up and down to find paper for the printer, new ink cartridges, pens, or sticky notes. Remind the members of your household that they need to respect your workspace.

Rise and Shine

Did you know that working remotely is not some form of vacation? I know that this is shocking news, but it is the truth. I have spoken to many remote workers who have told me that the most common misconceptions are that they don't have regular working hours. Another misconception is that they can sleep in every day and work in their pajamas. It may be hard to believe, but remote workers have schedules and deadlines that they need to stick to.

Wake up early and get yourself ready for the day while the coffee is brewing. Create a daily to-do list that includes everything you want to accomplish for the day. Send your schedule to your employer so that they know what your intentions are for the day. Most workplaces have a policy that prohibits employees from being active on social media platforms during working hours—maintain that policy. Social media is more distracting than the dogs barking or children asking for snacks.

Facing Challenges

Working from home is going to come with baggage that will test you, and it may even try to break you. It is not easy transitioning from working away from home to spending all your time at home. This is all related to changes, and we have established how people respond to those—not as well as could be expected. It is important to set up boundaries between your work and home life. Stick to office hours as much as possible, and don't allow your peers to bully you into working longer hours (unless you are being compensated). Your mental health and well-being need to be disciplined. Stick to the schedules you have created. Face your challenges like the champion that you are and rise to the occasion.

Setting Yourself up for Success

I spoke to a friend who woke up one morning to find that they were snowed in. They told me that thirty-nine inches of snow had fallen overnight and that it was continuing when they tried to open their front door. They were informed by their office manager to follow their pandemic protocol for working from home. The protocol was that everyone needed to log into their Microsoft Team accounts so that their employers could see that they were "at work." The friend told me that it was an adjustment working from home after working in the office. They said that they had more structure at the office and all their work comforts to offer the support they needed to maintain the high level of productivity they were accustomed to. They said that if they had been given a choice, they would have put on their skis to get to work instead of spending time being distracted and finding a comfortable chair to sit on.

Working from home might seem like an adventure, especially when most remote companies tell you that you can work from any location in the world. The adventure runs its course when you realize that you have more aches and pains in places you never thought existed. No one tells you, when you first start out, that you need a comfortable chair to support your posture or that you need a proper desk and that your television dinner tray is not ideal. It is important to create a workspace that allows you to feel as if you are working in an office. Your overall mental and physical health and well-being will be eternally grateful that you have made changes to help you succeed. I want to share a couple of "must-haves" to set you up for success on your remote working journey.

Comfortable Work Chair

Many seasoned remote workers will tell you that it is incredibly important to spend a couple of extra dollars on an ergonomic work chair. It will offer your spine the support it needs to prevent future ailments. It is also a good investment for your back because you will spend many hours sitting in that chair.

Keyboard Setup

Another must-have is an ergonomic keyboard that will provide support for your wrists. I have spoken to a transcription worker who told me that it was important to have a keyboard that supports your hands and wrists. They said that another option would be to purchase a stand that could elevate the keyboard to ensure that your wrists don't rest on the desk. It is important to take care of your hands and wrists because any neglect could lead to individuals experiencing nerve damage that causes pins and needles and numbness in your fingers.

Essential Office Tools

You may be working from the comfort of your home, but you still have colleagues who rely on your input. Remote workers are normally scattered across the country or the world, but thanks to the age of digital technology, everyone can experience the office environment. You don't have to be a computer whiz to use the virtual tools that will unite you and your colleagues. Let's look at the tools that your virtual office needs to support and enhance your productivity:

Communication Tools: Microsoft Teams, Google Meet, Slack, Skype, or Zoom.

Project Management Tools: ProofHub, Hive, HubSpot, or Workzone.

Remote Access Tools: TeamViewer, AnyDesk, RemotePC, or Splashtop Business Access.

Virtual Assistants: Siri, Alexa, or Google Assistant.

Virtual Assistant Tools: A stable and secure internet, fiber, or wi-fi connection; a webcam, external hard drive, or flash drives; and a computer that is dedicated to the sole purpose of your work.

Additional Measures to Succeed When Working Remotely

You have free rein to deck out your workspace with whatever you feel will help you be comfortable and increase productivity. I don't tell you what you should or shouldn't be doing and what you need or don't need. I do give you suggestions, but essentially, it is your workspace, and you have to do what is right for you. I would like to end this chapter with a couple more tips that you may like to add or introduce to your workplace. Some of the tips would be practical, and others would be for aesthetics:

- Recreate Your Workspace: You may feel more comfortable working from home if you recreate your desk at the office.
- Spare Accessories: It is also a good idea to have spare charging cables for your digital devices or your laptop, extra drives, cartridges for the printer, external

keyboard, and mouse; you never know when you may need those spares.
- Desk: You can't keep working on your dinner tray.
- Desk Light: Install a globe that offers you a soft glow to create a calming and stress-reduction atmosphere in your workspace.
- Natural Lighting: Create your workspace in an area that offers natural light, as well as a well-ventilated area, to ensure that you are surrounded by fresh air.
- Plants: Consider adding a couple of potted plants to your workspace to help keep you calm and reduce unnecessary stress.

Adapting to the New Dynamics in the Workplace

We know that the uninvited guest, COVID-19, opened its suitcases and threw the contents across the world. Everyone was affected because the whole world shut down, and restrictions were put in place. The contents of those suitcases created major obstacles that we had to learn to adjust to and, eventually, overcome. Billions of people sat in uncertainty as they waited for news. Employers had to think about the future of their companies and businesses. The choices were either to shut down until the pandemic eased up (no one knew when that would be) or work from home for the unforeseeable future. It was a no-brainer that they decided to permit their employees to work from home. Most companies sent their employees computers, monitors, and whatever else they needed to carry on with their work, and others purchased new equipment.

While companies and most businesses could continue working, other businesses suffered losses that crippled them. Some industries didn't offer the option to work from home, such as cosmetologists, hairdressers, beauty salons, and restaurants that didn't offer fast food options. COVID-19 stole the livelihood of billions of individuals, but it also created opportunities for those who put their skills to good use.

I remember a colleague telling me about a freelance company that grew from having eighty people in May of 2020 and, as of January 2023, was standing at over 2,600 individuals offering an array of services. The creation of jobs for the world of telecommuters was becoming more popular than working in an environment where people weren't happy. Not everyone will, indeed, be happy. They will take whatever they can find, but it is important to remember that success will only find those who make peace with the circumstances that lead them to their new position. We walk in wisdom, "See then that you walk circumspectly, not as fools but as wise" (Ephesians 5:15, NKJV). We are to be very careful, then, how we live—not as unwise but as wise, "making the most of every opportunity" (Ephesians 5:16, NIV).

I have previously mentioned that working from home requires a lot of discipline. You may argue that you know what discipline is all about because you worked in an office where you were surrounded by colleagues. Let me be the first to tell you that you don't know discipline until you have adjusted to working from home. You don't have anyone but yourself to hold you accountable if you decide to sleep in for an extra hour or two. You may find it more comfortable to "go to work" in your pajamas or only wear a work shirt for your meetings. You may have a compulsion and think that because you work from home, you can have as many breaks as you want. You are staring at the tail end of discipline because you may have decided to change the way you approach your work. What happens when your employer tells you that you must go back to in-person work and be socially distanced from your colleagues? You just spent at least eight months being "self-employed" and now that freedom is being taken from you and reinforced with even stricter rules to keep everyone safe. Your lack of discipline while working remotely is going to affect your mental health; that, in turn, may see you resenting your new normal in-person work. You will be like a city broken into and left without walls (Proverbs 25:28).

Introducing Workplace Models

Employers and business owners were introduced to a whole new world as COVID-19 made its presence known. They had to create ideas and solutions to continue providing services to their customers and clients, as well as keeping their employees and members of staff employed. Business owners met with consultants and strategists to help explore solutions for the new world that they found themselves in. Working remotely was only part of the solution, but employers had to look to the future. No one knows when COVID-19 will pack its bags and leave our shores, and until such time, everyone puts on their creative thinking caps to prepare for "when it ends." Various models were introduced to keep businesses afloat and to give employees a light at the end of their dark tunnels.

I will share a couple of the most popular models in this section, but it is important to understand that workplace dynamics have changed. I err on the side of caution when I say that people between the ages of thirty-five through sixty had to grow up very quickly during the pandemic. Working remotely was a new concept for many, and with that came changes that may not have been received with wide-open arms—a topic that has been discussed in previous chapters. Growing up is not all that easy for someone who had a routine of waking up, getting ready, commuting to the office, and working with their colleagues for over twenty to thirty years. Learning to adapt to something new was not on their to-do list, but they knew that it was doable, and it was a case of accepting the ongoing challenge.

The Old New Normal Model

This model would see employees returning to their old normal. They would resume their nine-to-five working hours and bounce back into their old routines. Many may be happy to return to their old normal, but this model features modifications that must be followed. Office workers would have to maintain the government health officials' pandemic guidelines, which include social distancing and wearing face masks.

The Hybrid Model

This model is also referred to as the clubhouse. The hybrid model allows employees to return to their workplaces when they need to attend in-person meetings or when they need to collaborate with their co-workers. In-person visits to their offices allow for socializing and opportunities to get work done without feeling isolated. Employees are still required to be mindful of the restrictions and mandates. They get to return home after their in-person visit and start working on the tasks they received at their meeting.

Jack-in-the-Box Model

I find this model very interesting, as it offers employees a variety of opportunities to ensure productivity. We know that the pandemic changed the way we worked and lived. Everyone had a designated workspace in their place of employment, but then the unthinkable happened, and the pandemic turned our

Chapter 5: Adjusting to Your New Workplace in the Pandemic-Altered World

world upside down. Employees found themselves creating workspaces in their homes and adapting to the new conditions. As restrictions eased and mandates were lifted, employers opted to implement some changes that they believed would benefit their employees, as well as be beneficial to their productivity. Their new post-pandemic model would see employees returning to the office, but instead of working from their desks, they would have the opportunity to work in various hubs around the office. These hubs could be the breakroom, the conference or meeting room, the lounge, or any space where you can do what you need to do but also work from home a couple of days a week.

I believe that this model was created with the health and well-being of employees in mind. Individuals with certain comorbidities were cautioned to self-isolate, and others were told they needed to exercise. The Jack-in-the-box model gave employers a little gap that they kicked wide open to implement in their workplaces so that employees could be active.

The Satellite Office Model

This model is very thoughtful and shows employees that their employers understand their struggles relating to commuting. I believe that this model may grow in popularity, even when the pandemic fizzles out one day. The jest of this model is to create smaller offices in various areas surrounding the main, centralized office in the heart of the city. Some employees may see themselves converting their garages or basements into office space where they can create satellite offices for their co-workers. This is a solution that may benefit many employees who get to work together in person, as well as be economically sustainable by saving on commuting. Thinking about the economic side of things, I really love this model—everyone wants to save money in this volatile economic climate.

Virtual Reality Model

This model has been spoken about, referred to, and discussed in great length. You either love the idea of working remotely, or you hate it. We know that we can't please everyone, but the reality is that businesses need to create practical means to keep their heads above water. We are living in a volatile economic climate that can claim the life of a business in a matter of days. Businesses have learned how to adapt to the pandemic, so why not put that knowledge to work and find ways to potentially save your company and cut down on costs? The virtual reality model gives employers that opportunity by having their employees work from home, the coffee shop, the library, or on the beaches of Hawaii. Business owners can sell their offices or give up their leases to save money. This model is a win-win for business owners and employees who have learned to embrace working remotely.

Adopting Workplace Dynamics for the Future

I recently spoke to someone who shared their thoughts and understanding of what the future of a pandemic-altered world reminded them of. They remembered watching reruns of *Star Trek*, when William Shatner played the role of Admiral James T. Kirk and Leonard Nimoy portrayed Commander Spock in the original television series that ran from 1966 to 1969 (*Star Trek*, 2023). They also remembered another show that offered a glimpse into the future—*The Six Million Dollar Man*—in which Lee Majors was the main character, Steve Austin (*The Six Million Dollar Man*, 2023). The series was on the air from 1973 to 1978. Both series offered a glimpse into the future, and nobody would have given it much thought if they hadn't watched reruns between the '70s and '80s. My interviewee said that they were transported back in time when the news of the pandemic broke, and their memories of the television shows resonated with what was happening. The only thing that they haven't discovered just yet is how to get cars to fly.

Maybe these shows, which were created over fifty years ago, were a prophecy of what the current world would look like. The world has evolved in more ways than we can think of because it is ever-changing. We must keep up or risk being knocked down at every obstacle that comes our way. The pandemic committed major crimes against humanity, such as affecting the physical health of billions, job losses, the loss of lives, and anger and hatred towards others. This is a list that will continue growing until COVID-19 and all its variants are sent packing to the Bermuda Triangle for an eternity. The future starts with us and what we can do to create our real-life futuristic series that plays out in real-time. A plan for prosperity and not to harm, plans of hope and a great future (Jeremiah 29:11), and forgetting the former things, not dwelling on the past.

The Benefits of the Hybrid Model

This is a fifty-fifty model that allows employees to work from home as well as in person. Most employees enjoy the choice and will split their time between the two workplaces. The hybrid model has benefits for both employers and employees. The biggest benefit for employees is that it reduces the costs involved in commuting. There is also the fact that employees don't face the risk of getting stuck in traffic, which wastes unnecessary time and results in a loss of productivity. I don't want to be a buzzkill, but remember that the freedom of working from home comes with responsibility. Employers will also benefit from utilizing the hybrid model. They can look forward to a reduction in business expenses, such as using less power, office supplies, and less telecommunication. Another benefit for employers is that they will have a staff that will be happy to work because they are given the freedom to work independently.

Connecting Technology and Humans

Virtual reality taught us that we could perform away from our workplaces. We were equipped with all the tools that required us to work independently and virtually. This was the marriage of technology and humans. Technology, love it or hate it, is integrated into our daily lives. We need it to stay connected to the outside world; without it, we are off course. I find it fascinating that we are in a place where *The Six Million Dollar Man* series is happening before our eyes. Artificial intelligence (AI) is an intimidating integration into our lives. I know of many people who have expressed their fear and what this collaboration would mean to their jobs. I have spoken to people who are well-versed in AI, and they have explained that the human touch will always be needed. It is part of our human nature to worry about all the changes that are happening, and listening to the doomsday chanters spreading fear is not helping or doing anyone any good. AI technology needs its human counterparts to build the resources it needs. It is believed that the relationship between the two will be a positive addition to health care, education, and getting supplies to their locations during a crisis.

A Gig-Based Employment Market

We saw the world implode because of the pandemic, but we also witnessed something that tickled the curiosity of many. The introduction—or should we say the reintroduction—of working remotely opened a branch of job opportunities for people who were struggling to get work. I spoke to a seasoned remote worker who told me that finding at-home jobs was extremely difficult before the pandemic. They said that, at the time, it felt as if they were digging around in illegal websites and forums to find legitimate opportunities to work from home. Scammers were preying on the vulnerabilities of people who wanted to work, and they were "offering" exorbitant amounts of money as payment, but first—here is the first sign that this is not an authentic opportunity—you had to pay for training materials and initiation costs. People fell for these scams because they were desperate. Always remember that a real company will not ask you for payments to use their resources for training.

The pandemic opened the doors to job seekers and talent hunters, who posted countless job opportunities on recruitment platforms, such as LinkedIn. This led to a new generation of people working remotely and brought about a shift in employment opportunities. Many companies decided that it would be better and more cost-efficient to build up a team of gig workers with varied talents, such as content creators, social media managers, narrators, editors, or freelance writers. These gig workers would be employed on a contract basis. It also allowed those who were freelancing to explore the job market and take on multiple tasks with other companies. Building up a pool of gig workers would also be beneficial to companies because they save on overhead expenses and other office-related costs.

Real-Life Adjustments

You may have anticipated being intimidated and afraid of the changes that would accompany the introduction of working remotely. This chapter has a lot of information that explains everything that you need to know to help you be a successful telecommuter. I know that people say that it is easy to transition to working from home, but it is something that not everyone wants or needs. I understand that you may want to be with people and have intelligent (or not-so-intelligent) conversations with your co-workers. You were forced to adapt to these changes or risk losing your job, especially when you live with someone who is labeled as medically fragile.

I spoke to someone who was forced to work from home, whether it was an option or not, when COVID-19 arrived. They said that the beginning of March 2020 saw them converting a space in their bedroom into an office by building a cubicle. They said that they didn't want to see their computer or workspace from their bed, and as they shared a house with their elderly parents, it was the best solution for them. The first couple of months were difficult, but they did what had to be done. The weeks turned into months, and they hadn't seen their friends for close to a year because they knew it was their responsibility to keep their elderly parents safe.

Their mental health was being affected, as they were the caregiver of their parents, and it was their duty to ensure that the parents remained safe. The restrictions started easing, and their parents were becoming restless and felt the need to go and do their own shopping and see what the world outside of their house looked like. My interviewee realized, at that point, that the pandemic had caused irreparable damage to the mental health of their parents. They blamed the pandemic as much as they did themselves for being over-protective, and they knew that they had to loosen the reins. The family was devastated when, for the first time in two years, the father went to the pharmacy to pick up medication and was exposed to the Coronavirus; he ended up in the hospital a couple of days later.

Chapter 5: Adjusting to Your New Workplace in the Pandemic-Altered World

Life throws all types of curve balls your way, and you can't always hit them. You must make tough decisions, and you must release the grip you have on certain situations. I know that the guilt that this comes with is real, but you can't blame yourself for a virus that has no boundaries and disregards personal space. The pandemic gave you many options, and one of those was so that you could retain your income by working from home. The next chapter is going to be about easing you back into in-person work and how to create a healthy work-and-life balance to rebuild and improve your emotional health. I will also include a helpful section on how to find a job during these difficult times. One. Two. Three. And we jump!

CHAPTER 6:

Putting the Pieces of Your Pandemic-Altered Work Life Back Together

"Do not remember the former things, Nor consider the things of old"

(Isaiah 43:18, NKJV).

"The secret of change is to focus all your energy not on fighting the old, but on building the new"

(Dan Millman).

I went to Target a couple of months ago and purchased a five-thousand-piece puzzle from the sale section. The box was a little tattered and worn, but the puzzle pieces were safe and secure in their plastic packaging. I continued with my shopping, went home, and unpacked my groceries. I made myself a cup of tea and sat down to inspect the box cover of the puzzle I had purchased. It was a breathtakingly beautiful sunrise over the ocean. The colors were bright and vibrant and made me feel that if I touched the cover, I would be magically teleported to the destination. Then, I noticed the parts of the cover that were faded and damaged, and I was overcome with sadness. This was a reminder of what COVID-19 had brought into our lives.

The pandemic changed the way we lived. You may argue that you didn't experience a life of laughter, brightness, and happiness—but you had freedom. You could go where you wanted without being told to do this, that, and the other. You didn't have anyone reminding you that you had restrictions. I certainly didn't have someone telling me to wear a face mask or spray sanitizer on my hands any time I went into a store. I also didn't have people scattering, as if I had done the abominable when I sneezed or coughed because of an irritating tickle. You cannot argue that we had a great life before COVID-19. The damage started at the end of December 2019, and it didn't take long for life as we knew it—the carefree days—to fade.

I look around now, and briefly, everything might be returning to the way it once was, but it will never be the same as it was pre-2019. I sense a lot of fright, and I can see that people are wary when they go somewhere or do something. We spend a lot of time thinking about the what-ifs when going to a public place, taking the children to the indoor play park, or being invited to parties or events. The optimist in me wants to shout

out that everyone will be fine, but the Debbie Downer in me wants to be cautious because I don't know if and when the next variant of the Coronavirus will rear its ugly little head. Do we throw caution to the wind, carry on with life, and worry about the consequences if and when they occur? This is one of those personal choice options where you must do what is best for you. All I can say, from my side, is that my mental health has been screaming, throwing tantrums, and pulling my hair out to live outside the forged cage I have built around myself. The fear of man lays a snare, but whoever trusts in the Lord will not fear; he shall not be moved. He shall be helped just at the break of dawn (Psalm 46:1–5). God provides safety to those who trust in Him so that He will be glorified (Ezekiel 28:26).

We were the cover of that puzzle box before COVID-19 arrived, with its suitcase full of destruction. The pandemic went from person to person—who unknowingly took it to another town, city, county, or country—and we watched it spread like wildfire. We became the damaged and faded part of that puzzle box; we became faded and damaged as the pandemic spread like wildfire. We didn't know what it would mean for us. The box may have been damaged and faded in most parts, but the plastic packaging on the inside was still sealed, and the puzzle pieces were protected. All that needs to be done is to open the packet and start putting the pieces together to recreate the picture on the cover. That is where we are today: learning how to recreate the picture. Our exteriors may have been defaced being patient in affliction, but we are joyful in hope; we have what it takes to build something new (Romans 12:12).

This chapter is all about putting the pieces of our work life back together after months of uncertainty. We didn't know if we would see the next day, let alone wonder whether we would ever return to normal. Telecommuting, or working remotely, presented temporary and permanent solutions for billions of employees. We all knew that the time would come when working arrangements would be reverted to in-person. Many employees became anxious at the thought of getting used to the traffic on their daily commute. Others didn't want to be in a situation where they were under scrutiny from their co-workers. Everyone has their reasons for being afraid of returning to the workplace, and that is what this chapter wants to help you with. I am going to share some tips to help ease you back into returning to in-person work, and I will also share some tips about helping you balance your work and life.

Easing Your Way Back to Working at the Office

The buzzing of the alarm clock is forcing you to regain consciousness. Your first reaction is to slap that snooze button into another hemisphere, but then you realize that you must get up and get ready for…work! This is not the same work routine that you have been following for the last eighteen or so months. You could wake up a little later, roll out of bed, put on the coffee maker, turn on the computer, finish getting dressed, and prepare for your workday. Not anymore, because you are headed off to the office for the first time in more than a year. You have been summoned, and re-enlistment to an office setting is going to happen, whether you are ready or not.

I know that a lot of people were excited about returning to in-person work, and even with restrictions and mask mandates still securely in place, they jumped at the opportunity. The introverts are a little more insecure about the changes because they have enjoyed working in solitude. They are also the type of people who prefer the simplicity of the routine that they have created

Chapter 6: Putting the Pieces of Your Pandemic-Altered Work Life Back Together

for themselves. Many of us learned to despise the pandemic for what it was doing, but there were some positives. One of those positives, in my eyes, was that it shook us out of our comfort zones. We get so used to following the same routine—day in and day out—that we get comfortable in our grooves. The pandemic shook us to our very cores, filled us with fear, and changed all the rules of life as we knew it.

I would like to make it clear that I am not here to force anyone to have the vaccine. I will also not be an advocate for or against it because, again, it is a personal choice that everyone must make for themselves. I don't entertain conspiracy theorists, and I also do not buy into the religiosity and political agendas that accompany the vaccine. We are all adults who should give others the freedom to make their own choices. I have seen friendships end and arguments start when people have the vaccine, and I don't want you to stop reading this because you believe I have a hidden agenda. It was only a matter of time before someone, or many someone, worked together to find a way to develop ways to strengthen immunity. The vaccines, regardless of personal opinions, may have given some employees the solution they required to return to a brand-new normal. Adjusting to that brand-new normal was not, and most likely will not be, as easy as everyone believed.

One day, you were working in your office. The next day, you were told that your country was going into lockdown and that you would be confined to your home. A few days down the line—after you've baked enough sourdough bread and banana loaves to start a bakery—you start to worry about your future. A couple of weeks into lockdown, your employer gives you two options, and you choose the one to work remotely. A year and a half later, you are informed that your pandemic-working vacation—working remotely—has been terminated and that you will be returning to in-person work. This is the scenario that just about sums up the last couple of years of your pandemic-led life. This is where you open the package with the puzzle pieces and start putting them together. The transition may not be easy, and it might take you a while to adjust, but the pieces of the puzzle will fit together to create a brand-new, brightly untarnished picture.

Adjusting to Your Brand-New Normal Work-Life

I don't know about you, but I am not a clairvoyant, and I don't know what the future holds. It is safe to say that no one knows what tomorrow will bring because every morning, when you open your eyes, is a new day waiting to be experienced. I have previously mentioned that everyone has a choice. You could choose to give up, or you could choose to adjust. I am, as you know, an eternal optimist—and giving up is not something you will find in my vocabulary. So, like me, choose to adjust. Look up to the hills for those great promises of His (Exodus 23:26), promises of protection, provisions not only in materials but also in health (Jeremiah 29:11). Our hope for tomorrow is not because of our righteousness but because we are in Him. The pandemic affected people in many ways, and it changed, and continues to change, the rules. The restrictions may have eased, allowing more freedom, but it will always be something we think about when going to the mall, the gym, a fast-food restaurant, any crowded venue, or your workplace.

The return to in-person work caused anxiety among many people—especially those who have children, medically compromised family members, or the fear of colleagues not respecting their boundaries. This pandemic business is new to everyone, and we all must learn by trial and error. I spoke to someone

Chapter 6: Putting the Pieces of Your Pandemic-Altered Work Life Back Together

who cocooned their little family into a bubble. They took all the measures to stay safe because they had a three-year-old, and their partner was a type-2 diabetic; it was important that the Coronavirus stay outside and as far away from them as possible. The day arrived when they were given notice that in-person work would resume. They took every possible precaution to ensure that they were safe by setting boundaries for their co-workers, wearing their face masks, and using gloves when dealing with orders. The measures that they took to keep their family safe knew no end. Their daily ritual included stripping down before they went inside, putting their clothes in the washing machine, and showering before greeting their family. The sad reality is that one person taking all the precautions to be safe and stay protected is not going to stop a herd of elephants from causing a stampede. It was only a matter of time before they were diagnosed with the Coronavirus, which then ricocheted, and everyone in the home was infected. Their partner ended up in the hospital and struggled because of severe scarring on their lungs.

The health side of returning to in-person work is one of many stepping stones. These stepping stones have allowed you to procrastinate about transitioning from remote working to in-person working. We have spent the better part of two years creating a work schedule that worked for us and your families. We may not have embraced the initial pandemic changes, but we learned to make it work to our advantage. We knew that we would return to "normal" if and when the spread of the virus slowed down. The time has arrived when I fly in on my unicorn to help you adjust and alleviate your anxiety. Grab a handful of glitter and use it to spread positivity as you adjust to being back in your office, where you are surrounded by your colleagues.

The Art of Compassion

I am always telling people that they should be kind to themselves. Colossians 3:12 (NIV) advises us specifically to "clothe yourselves with compassion, kindness, humility, gentleness and patience." Everyone deserves compassion because no one knows what someone else is going through. I read an article in which Dr. Meag-gan O'Reilly, a licensed psychologist, mentions that the swift and sudden changes and transition from office to home were negative for most people (Goodchild, 2021). The psychological side effects included uncertainty about what the future holds and the unprecedented loss and grief experienced. Doctor O'Reilly also mentions that remote workers may have initially set high expectations for themselves when they transitioned because they didn't have the structure or routines that they were used to, and other employees may find themselves struggling to focus.

Doctor O'Reilly ends off by saying that we spent the better part of two years relying on virtual communication. Employers and colleagues saw pets making themselves comfortable on laps or children running around or playing quietly in the background. The scenes that everyone got to see (and hear) allowed others to see the relaxed and human side of their colleagues. Always be kind to yourself and show compassion to yourself and your colleagues because I can assure you that everyone is feeling the side effects of the transitions they have had to endure over the last couple of years (Goodchild, 2021).

Establishing New Routines

The days of rolling out of bed ten minutes before you are due to start are coming to an end. You may want to rekindle your relationship with some pre-pandemic habits or create a brand-new routine based on all you learned while working remotely.

Start by preparing for your day the night before. Ensure that your work clothes are set out and that everything is ready for you—try and avoid the last-minute, early morning crisis that involves an iron or the need for a sewing kit. Meal-prepping breakfast, lunch, and dinner will become your saving grace as you and your new routine become best friends. Allow your routine to make provision for any commuting snags; remind yourself that you haven't had to deal with traffic and the ups and downs of commuting for a couple of years.

Setting Boundaries in the Workplace

Working remotely afforded you the flexibility of being lenient with your work hours. Returning to in-person work means that you don't give your employers or colleagues that same flexibility. You have set working hours that need to be adhered to—which means not contacting you after hours. Everyone, regardless of who they are, needs to have boundaries in place. It is beneficial for your mental and physical well-being. We don't want to create a doormat scenario where you are available at all hours of the day. Don't ever feel bad for using a certain two-letter word that others love to use, but never expect it to come from your mouth. Let's say it together—no. Maybe a little louder—no. Okay, one more time for good measure so that your neighbors can hear that you mean business—*no!*

Learning How to Create a Healthy Work-Life Balance

It may take you a while to find your routine, but I have confidence that you can do anything you put your mind to. Remind yourself that you can do hard things. Remind yourself that up until the moment that you are reading this, and every day after, you are a COVID-19 survivor. You may be tattered, torn, and a little weary, but you are a survivor. Change is never easy, but you did what you had to. I have previously referred to the older generation as being afraid of changes, but it doesn't mean that those who are twenty through forty years of age don't suffer anxiety, too. We lived in uncertainty, and we had entered that fight-or-flight mode where we knew that tomorrow may not be assured. We know that the Coronavirus didn't care about boundaries; we watched as our family, friends, and even strangers struggled when they were ill or when they experienced a loss.

I recently had someone tell me that the Coronavirus may have skipped their home, but it didn't mean that it didn't wreak havoc when a loved one had a heart attack or a stroke. The patients are left alone and often passed without anyone at their bedside. New parents were also affected because many hospitals would not allow the new father to be at the birth of their baby, nor were they allowed at any of the prenatal appointments. The point I am trying to get across is that it took COVID-19 to show us how precious life is and to learn how to prioritize our real lives. All it takes is a shift in your mindset and guidance to help you create a smooth and seamless work-life balance. A quick reference to the quote by Herophilus, a Greek physician, "When health is absent, wisdom cannot reveal itself, art cannot manifest, strength cannot fight, wealth becomes useless, and intelligence cannot be applied." This is very instructive. Safeguarding your health not only physically but also spiritually will allow you to fulfill your purposes (3 John 1:2), as well as enjoy abundant peace and security (Jeremiah 33:6).

Understanding Work-Life Balance

Having a work-life balance would ideally indicate that you spend half of your time focusing on your professional career and the other half keeping your personal life happy. I did say "ideally" because we all know that that is what we desire. How would you know if you aren't meeting the requirements of a perfect work-life balance? This section of the chapter is not to be seen as shining the light on anyone's professional or personal life. Let's look at a couple of examples that may lean toward your work life being unbalanced:

Taking your responsibilities at work seriously, and they cross the boundaries you have established. Spending more time than necessary at the office. Employing people to take care of personal responsibilities: nannies, babysitters, or cleaning or cooking services.

It is important to your overall mental and physical well-being that you have a healthy balance between your life and your work. The benefits of a healthy work-life balance include a reduction in stress levels, the prevention of burning out, and overall happiness. Chapter 5 saw various models that would play a positive role in your work-life balance. Take your proposal to your employer and remind them that you had been working from home for several months. Explain that you were relying on outside help to raise your children, whereas, during lockdown, you were working and managing to raise your children without affecting your productivity. You will not know if they will agree with your suggestion if you don't take a chance and ask them.

We spend so much time trying to please our employers and colleagues because we believe that they need us. If you have learned anything from the pandemic, it is that you need to prioritize yourself. You had to make changes and sacrifices—just like everyone else. You had to adjust—just like everyone else. Your health and well-being were being tested—yes, you've got it, just like everyone else. You are putting your life on the line by prioritizing everyone first. Stop! Re-evaluate your needs. Do what is right for yourself and set those boundaries. What do we make of the word of wisdom in Ecclesiastes 4:6 (NKJV), "Better a handful with quietness Than both hands full, together with toil and gasping for the wind"? We should create a healthy balance between our active life and sedentary life. Safeguarding our health will allow us to fulfill our divine potential and relate with others more effectively.

Always remember that your happiness is important. You won't find that work-life balance if you are not happy in your career. Find a job that ticks all the boxes on your scale of happiness. Find a job that excites you and makes you want to go to work with a song in your heart and a smile on your face. Do your obligations outweigh your happiness? Do you believe your family will be content with someone who is grouchy or showing signs of depression? You will meet your work-life balance goals if you are doing something you love. Let's look at some helpful ways in which you can create the healthy work-life balance that you deserve:

Perfection is overrated: Don't compare yourself to others who say that they spend an equal amount of time at work and with their families; do the best you can by having realistic goals and doing what is needed to create a balance that works for your profession and personal life.

Don't neglect your health: It is vitally important that you find a career path that doesn't affect your health or cause you to experience the boomerang effect because you are unhappy; work-life balance, your health, and your happiness are the important ingredients to set you up for healing in mind, body, and soul.

Ditch those screens: Turn off your phone the moment you walk into your home; it's okay to use that all-important boundary that lets your employers and colleagues know that you have set working hours.

Self-care: This is one of my favorites because it allows you to schedule time for yourself and your loved ones to spend time together; nothing is more revitalizing for the mind and body than focusing all your attention, love, and joy on your loved ones. Be wise in the way you act towards outsiders, and make the most of every opportunity (Colossians 4:5).

Job Hunting in A Pandemic-Altered World

I have found that most people are in careers they are not passionate about. When asked why they are doing the work they are doing, many responses will be along the lines of, "My father was this, my mother was that," "You can make more money," or "That was all I could find." I have also interviewed a lot of people who didn't hold back with their responses and shared that their parents would only support them if they followed a career path that their parents chose.

One of my interviewees told me that they went through a difficult time during their teenage years. They had health problems that had stunted their growth, and with that came a lot of bullying, which affected their mental health. They started doing things that they shouldn't have been doing, which included self-harming, drinking alcohol, and using narcotics. They didn't have anyone to talk to other than their nanny, who had taken care of them since the age of three. It was also a case where the parents didn't have a work-life balance and entrusted their children to the nanny—who took them to school, went to doctor's appointments, and did everything a parent should have been doing. My interviewee didn't complete their schooling and dropped out at the end of grade eleven. They tried to find work and were willing to do anything to earn an income, but each of the jobs was temporary. They responded to an advertisement looking for volunteers to help take care of and train shelter dogs—fulfilling a dream of working with animals. Their parents were devastated. Ten years later, they were earning a salary doing something they felt passionate about: training service dogs for individuals with diabetes, seizures, and several other types of medical disabilities.

I'm not telling you to quit your job, but I am saying that you need to think of your happiness. We have been given the power to make choices regarding our ultimate destiny. Made bad choices? There are always second, third, fourth, and unlimited chances for a re-evaluation. Turn your mess into beauty and use it for your own good. It is debilitating to be in a job that you don't enjoy. It can, and most likely will, affect your mental health because you will feel trapped, angry, or frustrated. Eventually, your negative feelings will spill over, and your physical health will begin to decline. Make the choice that is right for you.

We know that COVID-19 came into our lives with the intention of turning everything upside down. It shook us to the core, and we had to learn how to crawl before we could walk and walk before we could run again. Everything that we knew and believed in had to be re-evaluated. I saw a lot of people doubting themselves, and others worrying about what the next day would bring. Many people joined the unemployment lines, as companies and businesses were closed indefinitely. Health protocols had to be figured out, and many people relied on their income to keep the roof over their heads, food on the table, and power to keep the lights on. Here is a million-and-one-dollar question: How do you find a job during and after a pandemic?

The million-and-two-dollar answer to your question is to follow me as we explore some helpful advice to set you up for success.

Free Courses

The internet, and most especially the University of Google, has a knowledge database of hundreds of websites that offer free up-skilling courses. Reputable websites such as LinkedIn, Coursera, or edX offer free and reasonably affordable courses. Visit the local education institutions in your community to sign up for any free course they may be offering. No one is telling you that you must work in the field you are doing courses in, but they are excellent building blocks to help you expand your knowledge base and grow your skills. The days of sitting around and waiting for something to fall from the sky are long gone, and you need to find ways to empower yourself. Be full of positivity, energy, and new ideas; for you have not been given the spirit of fear but of power, and love, and of a sound mind (2 Timothy 1:7), and whatever you do, work at it with all your heart (Colossians 3:23). Job hunting is challenging. I have spoken to individuals who have said that when they look at the requirements for a particular job listing, they don't qualify or don't have the necessary skills. This is where I tell them to take those requirements and use them to search for courses or tools that will build the arsenal they need to fulfill the skills they need. Don't let the job listings and their requirements intimidate you. Build your curriculum vitae (CV) and list all the courses you have done. Potential employers will see that you are showing passion and the desire to learn.

Volunteering

Are you currently unemployed?

Are you actively looking for a job?

I would suggest that you volunteer your services at various organizations in your community if you have answered yes to these questions. I have clients who have said they sit around the house or hang out with friends because they don't have a job. Many have said that they are emotionally drained because of all the unsuccessful applications. My solution is to use your time doing something in your community that you are passionate about. If you enjoy working with the older generation, find a nursing home or a pastoral care center where your services will be appreciated. This could include reading, washing their hair, giving manicures, or just having lively conversations. If you are passionate about animals, find a shelter and spend time at the facility while cleaning up the cages, bathing the dogs, grooming cats, or playing with them. Who knows, you may end up like the person who made a career out of training animals to be caregivers for people.

I know that offering your services for free is not popular in the current economic climate. Volunteers don't get paid, but you will acquire the necessary skills to fill the requirements of job listings. What better way to learn new skills than by being of service to organizations that will appreciate the help and time? You may even be one of the lucky ones who will be offered the opportunity to go to nursing school or enroll in the courses you need to be a teacher at a play school at the expense of the organization. You will never know what opportunities are waiting if you don't take that all-important first step. Volunteering is part of God's design for all. "A generous person will prosper; whoever refreshes others will be refreshed" (Proverbs 11:25, NIV). Also, if you "spend yourselves in behalf of the hungry and satisfy the needs of the oppressed, then your light will rise in the darkness, and your night will become like the noonday" (Isaiah 58:10, NIV).

Chapter 6: Putting the Pieces of Your Pandemic-Altered Work Life Back Together

We can't blame all our problems on COVID-19. It is easy to play this blame game, but we should be held accountable, too. The pandemic was, and is, being used as a scapegoat for many of the problems we are facing today, which include unemployment, crime, and poverty. I have previously said that every morning when we wake up, we have choices. Each choice has options or consequences. You can choose to stay in bed the whole day, but then you shouldn't blame your unemployment status on anyone else. Wake up every morning and say that you are going to have a great day. Get yourself ready, print out your curriculum vitae, and visit businesses or stores. Have a positive attitude and use the tools this chapter has presented you with to sell yourself to potential employers. Show people who you are and what value you can add to their business. This is the opportunity that you need to take responsibility for yourself. We can't blame COVID-19 for everything that doesn't go according to plan.

Having a job will put you on the road to financial freedom. This is something that we will be looking at in the next chapters. The road to financial freedom is an educational process that you must relearn. The restrictions we experienced during the pandemic did affect the financial world in more ways than we realized. It took the world returning to a new normal, opening the borders, and growing businesses again to realize that we are in an economic crisis. We have watched as interest rates have been hiked, the cost of basic food has increased, and gas prices have reached an all-time high.

Let's look at what you can look forward to as we prepare to dive into the next chapter. The very first topic will find us looking at the financial damage that COVID-19 brought in its suitcase. This will be followed by tearing apart and analyzing our saving and spending habits. Don't despair because I will end the chapter with a helpful guide to show your wallet or bank account how to cope with the turbulent economic climate. Are you ready to dive into the treacherous waters of the financial world? Let's go!

CHAPTER 7:

Financial Insecurity in Your Pandemic-Altered World

Coronavirus has exposed for all what many of us already knew—some of our most important workers have barely enough to live on, and millions are condemned to financial insecurity, inequality and food poverty.

Caroline Lucas

I alluded to the financial concerns we find ourselves in as we try to put the pieces of our lives back together. I do believe that everyone defaulted to playing the blame game. I know of people who continue to play the blame game, and they have been informed that the excuses are wearing thin. The first two years of the pandemic saw consumers drowning under the mass of debt that they couldn't keep up with. Many of these people had lost their jobs without notice, and others tried to find work to afford the minimum payments due. In short, everyone was struggling to keep their heads above water because they were simply not receiving benefits and salaries. Few governments gave out stimulus checks to their citizens.

I did a little bit of snooping here and a great deal of sniffing there and found out that most financial institutions offered their clients short-term financial relief. Other financial institutions kicked the doors wide open and bombarded their customers with constant calls from debt collection agencies. The harassment caused unnecessary stress and anxiety and left individuals afraid of what their future would look like. I can tell you that if you haven't had the unfortunate pleasure of speaking to or dealing with debt collection agencies, you can consider yourself lucky. These people will intimidate you in any way, shape, or form that they see fit; it is as if they know your weaknesses.

I spoke to a lady who informed me that she had been a customer of a company for over twenty years. She used her store card to purchase food for herself and for others who needed some assistance. She found herself without a job when news of the pandemic and lockdown was announced. The lady did what every responsible consumer should have done: she contacted all the companies she had accounts with and informed them of her retrenchment. This large company refused to acknowledge the retrenchment correspondence. She had been paying insurance on her account since she received her store card. Insurance means that customers are covered in the event of being retrenched, illness, or death. It wasn't long after they refused to acknowledge the insurance claim that the debt collectors started calling. She informed them that the company refused to help her. She explained the situation to them, and they tried to help her until the overdue account was reallocated to another company who were informed not to believe "sob" stories. She makes minimum payments and doesn't really worry about the interest that gets added because the case is being investigated by the Consumer Council.

Billion-dollar financial organizations and companies, and even consumers, need to realize that no one invited COVID-19 to turn their lives upside down. The blame game is getting old, and the scapegoat needs to retire. Companies need to listen to their consumers and come up with a plan of action without intimidation; consumers need to retire the "get out of obligations card" and acknowledge their debt. We need to be responsible for our actions, and that is what this chapter is going to teach you. It is up to everyone to make the necessary changes, to start building a pathway that will eventually be their new road to financial freedom. This journey will help us to grow our financial seeds, redirect the pointing fingers of blame, and finally retire the pandemic scapegoat.

Your Journey to Financial Health and Well-Being

We don't realize that everything that happens in our lives affects our overall mental and physical health and well-being. We take on the role of the modern-day superhero, and sometimes to our detriment. I recently attended a focus group where a group of individuals was talking about their inability to set boundaries and how it affected them both mentally and physically because they were being taken advantage of by the people they loved and trusted. Half of the group acknowledged that their family and friends were preying on their weaknesses, and they weren't afraid to play mind games.

I reached out to some of my interviewees, who shared that they, too, were duped by people who knew their weaknesses.

I think it is time to take those superhero titles that you have created for yourself and burn them. Remember, without counsel, plans fail, but with many advisers, they succeed (Proverbs 15:22). You need to do what is beneficial to you. Stop falling for the sad sob stories that play on your heartstrings and pull you away from your financial goals. Time for another secret—so, come a little closer: everyone suffered through the employment and subsequent economic crisis during the pandemic. And guess what? Everyone, whether they want to admit it or not, is being affected by the current financial problems as interest hikes threaten our purse strings. I know that this is shocking news, but it is the reality we are experiencing.

A Glimpse into the Financial Future of a World in Crisis

The financial implications were evident when the world shut down, travel bans were put in place, and rules and regulations were enforced; jobs were in jeopardy, businesses were at risk of facing bankruptcy, and the outlook for the immediate future didn't look so bright. Businesses that offered essential services, such as grocery stores, thrived, while smaller businesses and non-essential services were forced to close their doors for the unforeseeable future. Thousands of people lost their jobs or accepted work at a reduced salary, which caused financial strain on their households.

Chapter 7: Financial Insecurity in Your Pandemic-Altered World

We all had to learn how to tighten the purse strings and become mindful of what we spent our money on. A group of social and demographic researchers put together a survey in 2021—a year into the pandemic—to find out how individuals were doing and to gain insight into their thoughts about the financial situation they were facing (Horowitz et al., 2021). It is believed that 44 percent of the target audience had high hopes that their finances would take about three to four years to recover to their pre-pandemic status. Of upper-income families, it was noted that 39 percent had shown improvement in their financial situation during the first year of the pandemic. Americans are believed to have seen an increase—from 47 percent in April 2020 to 53 percent in March 2021—in their personal financial situations.

The researchers discovered that approximately four in ten Americans spent less money during the first year of COVID-19. All income tiers have expressed that they were spending less because they were concerned about their personal finances. Everyone said that they were able to enforce the savings because their daily activities have been restructured. I believe that these income groups could save during that first year because money wasn't being spent on commuting, children weren't going to school, and the normal day-to-day expenses were cut in half (Horowitz et al., 2021).

The first year of the pandemic saw upper-, middle-, and lower-income groups do well in the financial department. We don't know what the future will look like. The researchers have put together a compilation of answers that were collected during their survey. Individuals weighed in with their predictions of what their financial future would look like. Fifty-one percent of individuals who are not retired have expressed that the pandemic will prevent them from reaching their financial goals for their golden years; a handful of individuals believe that it will be easier. At least forty-one percent have said that they don't know what the future holds. The consensus is that, indeed, we don't know what the future holds. We cannot predict what obstacles will jump up in the financial world to knock us off our new roads to finding financial freedom. Consider following some of the helpful tips that have been presented throughout this book to supplement your income and take on freelance work to improve your finances. This may be a temporary solution until you can find yourself looking towards the clouds to find the silver lining you have been waiting for. Remember that the pandemic won't last forever, and yes, the side effects may be felt for years to come, but you have the equipment to break the hold it has over you (Horowitz et al., 2021).

Spending and Saving Habits During a Global Pandemic

This is another one of those "be thankful for COVID-19" moments. The pandemic brought about destruction and devastation, but it also brought some positive aspects. It may have taken us a couple of years to see anything positive about the pandemic. It was only a matter of time before our patience was rewarded. COVID-19 forced us to slow down, and it also united families who were buckling under the pressures of work-life balance. I know that you can't please everyone, and many of my readers may not agree with my statements—that's okay. We are all allowed to have opinions, which include seeing the positive side of a negative situation. We need to make little tweaks here and there to make things work for us. All my books are written in a way that my readers can take suggestions, hints, or examples and tweak them to suit their situations. We shouldn't be afraid to make changes or get stuck in a rut with no escape plan.

Chapter 7: Financial Insecurity in Your Pandemic-Altered World

I have hinted at the "be thankful for COVID-19" moments in the previous section, where consumers acknowledged that their financial situations had improved during the first year of the pandemic. They were more aware of their money and knew that they had to turn every dollar over three times. I must admit that I found it easy to save during the first year of the pandemic because I didn't have to drive to work or buy beauty products, clothing, and shoes I would need for work. I also saved on going to the hairdresser once a month and started doing my own nails. I wasn't running to the store after work each day to purchase ready-made food, and I learned to shop for groceries once a week and make my own healthier meals.

Financial Hits and Misses

The statistics proved that many individuals saved during the first year of the pandemic, some even building up a pandemic nest egg. Others weren't as fortunate to have the extra money to save because they fell under the income bracket that was already living on the breadline. These individuals found themselves struggling to make ends meet and relied on help from charity and religious organizations to put food on their tables. I have spoken to people who have found themselves in these situations, and I have witnessed the embarrassment of having to ask for assistance.

One of my colleagues told me about a friend who was stubborn, independent, and would rather suffer before asking anyone for help. They said that they phoned their friend to find out how they were doing and immediately picked up that something was wrong. My colleague asked their friend, and the response was always the same—nothing. They pushed a little until the friend broke down in tears and said that they had turned their refrigerator off because it was using unnecessary electricity. My colleague was confused and eventually found out that their friend had no food, other than rice for their dogs, in their home. They had been without food for four days at that time. My colleague went out, bought groceries, and took them to their friend. The friend was embarrassed, in tears, and thankful for the help. This was, and is, the reality of COVID-19. Many people had money and jobs, and many others had nothing but a mountain of debt.

Consumers were invited to participate in various surveys to determine the saving and spending habits of the American population. One of the surveys determined that half the American population had less than $250 after paying debt and utilities each month (Tymkiw, 2022). Others were not so lucky, with a staggering 12 percent of the participants indicating that they had nothing or couldn't fulfill their financial obligations after paying their bills. We have determined that debt is a noose around most people's necks. Many individuals turned to their credit cards to help them cross hurdles, but it was a short-term solution for what would become a long-term problem. The survey concluded that 53 percent of the American population was negatively affected by the arrival of COVID-19.

Spending Money During a Pandemic

Pandemic rules and regulations started easing, and people were confident about resuming their pre-COVID-19 lives. The rate of positive infections was decreasing, which many attributed to the vaccine. This, in turn, opened a couple of crevices that individuals could crawl through to explore the "world of shopping" to their heart's content. Many consumers believed that their finances would have improved by the end of the second year of the pandemic. The National Retail Federation (NRF) shared figures of how much money American consumers spend, as well as a prediction of what the spending habits would look like as restrictions are eased (Inman, 2021). The NRF has indicated that consumers spent approximately $3.9 trillion in 2019 and $4 trillion in 2020. Their prediction for 2021 was that consumers would collectively have spent over $4.3 trillion.

These figures and predictions are not meant to be an open invitation for you, the consumer, to go out and spend every nickel you have in your bank account or purse. Economists have suggested that you build up a nest egg because you don't know what tomorrow may bring. Remember the saying? "There is treasure to be desired and oil in the dwelling of the wise; but a foolish man spendeth it up" (Proverbs 21:20, KJV). Set aside something now for unexpected events in the future. We were all witnesses to the early 2020 news reports of the world shutting down. We don't know what will happen in 2024 or 2030. Invest your money in savings bonds, hide it under the floorboards, or stuff it in your mattress. Set aside an amount each month, and then budget according to the money that is left. Always be prepared for the unknown.

Re-Evaluating Your Personal Financial Habits

The NRF and economists predicted that consumers would be resuming their spending habits with a vengeance. This is a case of money burning a hole in people's pockets. The invisible bars holding you hostage have been removed, and you are ready to barrel out of your bubble to rejoin the tithing into the retail coffers. This may be a slight exaggeration based on some levels of truth. You spent the better part of two years living like a miser and creating financial habits to help you cope with the possibility of losing your income. Most Americans were saving, and by the time the restrictions were eased, they had a substantial amount of money saved.

Consumers were, and are, being cautioned to show restraint when spending money. Economists have advised consumers to be mindful of their spending habits and would advise building up a nest egg that would see them live comfortably for a year. This is where we must work on our priorities and re-evaluate our spending habits. Can you think back to when you were younger and received money from the tooth fairy, Grandpa sneaking a dollar bill into your hand without anyone seeing, or getting paid for doing chores? What did you do, or want to do, with the money you had? Did you allow your parents to put it in a bank account, drop it into the piggy bank, or demand to go to the gas station to buy treats?

I reached out to a couple of my interviewees. I had them step back in time to remember what they did with their money. No one had bank accounts as children, but the closest was a piggy bank that only had an entry point and no exit. Less than half of my interviewees said that they were the "burning a hole in my pocket" type of child who needed to spend their money as soon as they got it. The others were saving for a rainy day. I reached out to a group of children between the ages of six and ten, and I asked them the same questions. The younger children were split between putting money in the piggy bank or demanding a gas station outing. The older children had bank accounts and preferred to save their pocket, birthday, confirmation, and special money to save up for something they wanted.

We find ourselves in a similar scenario today, except we are not children and, as adults, we have responsibilities. It is up to each of us to be responsible for our finances. I know how tempting it is to just throw caution to the wind and go on a spending spree, but that is not going to help us without financial security. A large part of our financial security is based on our habits and the choices we make. A wise man thinks ahead; a fool doesn't and even brags about it. "All who are prudent act with knowledge, but fools expose their folly" (Proverbs 13:16, NIV). Similarly, "The thoughts of the diligent tend only to plenteousness; but of every one that is hasty only to want" (Proverbs 21:5, KJV). It is wise for us to plan and think through how we will make money and spend money. I want to look at a couple of examples that you may have created or want to create to set yourself up for financial freedom. I am a huge fan of recycling goals and habits. We become used to the ones we have created, and they lose their effectiveness because we have figured out how to work around them. Recycling your goals and habits is one of the stepping stones that hold you accountable for your financial situation.

Habits for Consideration

This section is going to give you an idea of the types of habits you may want to keep, what no longer applies to you, and how to try something new. Remember that I am not an economist, so everything I am sharing is based on my personal experience or those of my interviewees.

Debt Busting

I had someone tell me that they don't normally like to buy items on credit but that it is sometimes necessary. They needed a kettle in an emergency, and they didn't have the cash to purchase another one. They ordered their new kettle, and each month, they paid an extra amount over and above what was required. This helped them to finish paying off their debt sooner than expected, which saved on interest. Another person told me that they would pay extra into running monthly accounts such as phone, gas, or utility bills. Paying a couple of dollars extra each month would result in a month where they could skip a payment. If you have mountains of debt, pay what you can afford on all your accounts, but choose one account to pay a little more until it has been settled. You can continue doing this until you have repaid all your debt. Repay your debt. "The wicked borrow and do not repay, but the righteous give generously" (Psalm 37:21, NIV).

Savings One-Oh-One

The days of employers handing over your weekly or monthly paycheck have been retired. Most employees have their money transferred into their bank accounts, and from there, it gets diverted to wherever it needs to go. A great way to save a portion of your paycheck is to open a separate account where you can invest your money. Transfer 5–10 percent of your paycheck into the account, and then continue to budget the remainder of your pay. You may find yourself tempted to use your savings but forget that you have a separate account. Start another account, put away twenty dollars a month, and use that as your savings account to buy luxury items. "All who are prudent act with knowledge" (Proverbs 13:16, NIV)

The Thrice-Turned Dollar

The first year of the pandemic put the fear of Scrooge McDuck into us, and we pinched those pennies and turned each dollar over three times before buying a bag of candy or splurging on taco meal kits at Costco. This is a habit you may want to hold onto and maybe tweak to be a little more lenient. Remember that the pandemic may not be entirely over, but it has allowed you to step out and experience some freedom.

Chapter 7: Financial Insecurity in Your Pandemic-Altered World

A Little

Your financial health does not expect or rely on you to have a boring life. Did you know that saving can become an obsession? This is a habit that has been inherited from grandparents. They would tell us stories about how they lived on rations during the World Wars and the Great Depression. We would be entertained with stories about bartering rations with neighbors or community members to have a special breakfast for someone's birthday. They would share that they didn't have much money, and whatever money they earned was saved. I dare to say that our older generation of family members was resourceful because they would offer their crafts and skills to get some coffee, sugar, or eggs. Saving became an obsession, and many of our grandparents and great-grandparents had more money than most individuals because of their creativity. I am here to tell you that you shouldn't be careless with your savings but that you should also live a life. "The wisdom of the prudent is to give thought to their ways, but the folly of fools is deception" (Proverbs 14:8, NIV). As long as you have enough money to survive for a year, book yourself a weekend or a family getaway. Provide for your household. God is honored when we are diligent, prudent, hardworking, as well as rich in good works.

Examples of Implementing New Habits

The list of possible habits is long, and everyone has their own way of doing things. I have found that people do not always welcome advice, which is why I don't force my opinions or thoughts onto anyone. Let's look at some examples of habits you may want to add to your personal financial arsenal:

Plan for taxes.

You may want to see whether you can refinance your loans.

Draw up a budget or reach out to a financial advisor for help.

Consider automating your finances so that your accounts are paid before you spend. A great move to pay back what we owe.

Assist where help is needed, whether financially or purchasing groceries—don't give something with the expectation of getting it back. Be rich in good works.

Creating Your Breaking-Free Budget

This chapter has covered everything that you may want to know about your financial health and well-being. It also includes a prospective outlook of what the future may hold for you. The most important parts of this chapter must be all the examples, hints, and tips to help you wade through your financial turmoil. I know that the future might not seem so bright for now, but remember the puzzle I purchased at Target? The box was damaged, but the pieces of the puzzle were protected and ready for me to build. Your personal financial outlook may not look too bright now, but you will get to your goal. Remember that everyone has found themselves in situations far worse, and they have survived their personal pandemics. Personally, I am greatly inspired by these two Bible teachings in Proverbs 21:5 (NKJV), "The plans of the diligent lead surely to plenty, But those of everyone who is hasty, surely to poverty." "But remember the LORD your God, for it is he who gives you the ability to produce wealth, and so confirms his covenant" (Deuteronomy 8:18, NIV).

I am reminded of a story that someone shared about their grandmother, and I enjoy a giggle each time I think about it. The grandmother had five children, and sadly, none of them got along—which meant that birthdays and holidays were divided into time slots, and each child with the family was allocated a time. The third son was a bit of a bragger and would flex his financial wealth to the grandmother, knowing that she would tell his siblings. He would boast about buying property to build houses; every year, he had a new car, and he went away on lavish vacations. The grandmother was talking to her youngest daughter and gossiping about her brother. The daughter told her mother to stop and think for a moment about where that money came from. The grandmother thought about it, and the answer wouldn't come to her until the next day.

She phoned her daughter. "That boy stole the money I had hidden in a secret panel in my closet!" she exclaimed as her daughter answered the phone. "I went to look, and it is empty!"

The daughter laughed and said, "Mommy, my brother has all this money because he used credit. Everything he owns is funded by banks and credit companies. And Mommy, that secret compartment has been empty for more than thirty years."

The brother who flexed his wealth has managed to turn his spending habits around, paid all the creditors, and lives a cash-in-hand lifestyle. This may be because two of his siblings have passed on, and he doesn't need to flex for his nieces because he doesn't acknowledge their existence. The point I am trying to get across is that we get sucked into a false life where we do stupid things to impress people or make them green with envy. If he had been living his lifestyle during the pandemic, he may just have found himself in a homeless shelter. "Dishonest money dwindles away, but whoever gathers money little by little makes it grow" (Proverbs 13:11, NIV).

The bars of your pandemic jail cell have been removed, and you are free to go back to work. You may be one of those who has been saving money during the pandemic. Restrictions and mandates have been eased and lifted, and you have received the news that you have to return to in-person work. Your heart starts looking for an escape route out of your chest, the blood drains from your head, and you start sweating ice cubes—your anxiety is off the charts. Your financial bubble has popped, and you now must start working on a budget to accommodate the expenses you haven't needed for the last two years. You may also want to look at a variety of alternatives.

Commuting Woes

The price of gas plays a huge role in your return to the new normal. Look into alternative methods, such as public transport or share carpooling. I can assure you that you are not the first, and you most definitely will not be the last, to cut down on transport costs.

Lunch Time

I'm not going to be the bearer of that harsh news and tell you that you can't enjoy that mouthwatering shrimp salad wrap at your favorite deli around the corner from your office. I am going to try to be the voice of reason and remind you that you have lived without eating at that deli for nearly two years. You may have saved approximately $300 a month—$300 that can be used elsewhere. You can save on work lunch expenses by cooking extra at dinner and enjoying leftovers for lunch. Enjoy lunches that have been budgeted for when shopping for the week's groceries. I'm not telling you that you can't have the shrimp salad wrap or any other favorite, but I am trying to help you see where you can save money.

Caffeine Fix

I do believe that coffee makers are a fixture in most homes. Some may have fancier pod machines, while others are still using the original ones that require filters and ground coffee beans. Not everyone will have a coffee maker, or personal preference may have individuals purchasing instant coffee which is as good as freshly brewed. During your remote working days during the pandemic, you relied on your coffee-making skills to kick-start your morning. There is nothing better than pouring that first cup of liquid gold into a mug, adding milk and sweetener, bringing the cup to your mouth, and inhaling the aroma just before taking a sip. The coffee hits the taste buds, explodes, and jumps around to all the nerves to let them know that their wait is over—the caffeine fix is on its way. This is something you may have been doing every day since you started working from home. The coffee used was part of your weekly or monthly shopping budget. You didn't have a Starbucks or Dunkin' Donuts in your home, and you survived. Fill your travel mug with your freshly made caffeine fix that has been budgeted for. Save your coffee shop caffeine fixes for special occasions. Wisdom dwells with prudence… (Proverb 8:12). They are never apart.

What about the Children?

You had to learn how to work or have meetings with your children—chasing the dog or screaming because their sibling took their treats—in the background. It wasn't only the adults who were forced to stay and work from home; schools and daycare facilities were closed, too. You saved a pretty penny by disenrolling your little children from daycare because you didn't want to spend money on something you were not going to utilize. Remember that no one knew when in-person schooling or work would be resuming to the new normal. You spent the better part of eighteen months working from home with your kids underfoot. You may have complained, but secretly, you enjoyed every moment because it brought you and your family closer. You watched them grow and thrive under your watchful eye. You became more involved in their lives, and that is something you will miss. The question you are left asking is whether you use the money you would have spent on daycare to employ a nanny. Your children will be the center of attention in the comfort of their homes. The nanny could take the children on outings, to extramural activities, and arrange play dates with other children. You have many other options that you could explore, which include grandparents, family members, friends, or back to daycare. Your budget for childcare may be more than any other item on your list, but I know that you will do anything for the happiness of your children.

Final Round-Up

This chapter has been insightful. I am constantly reminded that no one knows what someone else is going through. The story about my colleague and their friend who didn't have food or money really touched my heart. I know that the friend was taking on odd jobs and relied on commission and gratuities to keep food in their refrigerator. The last I heard was that they are in the process of training for a job where they can work remotely, have freedom, and be paid a proper fixed income without worrying too much.

I wanted to end this book with a chapter that may be slightly heavier than the other topics we have covered. Talking about finances is not an easy topic, especially if you are not a financial advisor or an economist, but it is important to acknowledge the nooses around people's necks. I have always tried to avoid

Chapter 7: Financial Insecurity in Your Pandemic-Altered World

talking about money, and I know many people who feel this way because they believe that someone will ask them for a handout. I might have felt that way, too, but my eyes have been opened, and I can see when people are too proud to ask for help. I have learned to read people, and it is a humbling experience to get to know these individuals who would rather give than take anything.

I recently had a client who was going through more than they could cope with. Their financial situation had never been stable, and they found themselves at the receiving end of some massive mountains of debt. They didn't want to trouble their partner with what was happening in their financial bubble. The partner found out about the financial challenges and never wanted to be part of it because they believed that it was too messy and not part of their responsibility to pay the rent, pay school fees, or even purchase food. My client fought a noble battle until their world crumbled to pieces around them. The partner found out about the development, ended their relationship, took their dog, and removed their child. The turn of events and the sudden break-up caused my client—who is a self-harmer—immense mental trauma. They knew that harming themselves would lead to them never seeing their child, and the next best thing was to reach out to whoever they could for advice to turn their life around as quickly as possible. Solutions, advice, and even financial help flooded in. In a matter of three weeks, they were settled into a new apartment, and their debt was on the way to being sorted out. The only obstacle remaining is that the partner would not give my client permission to see their child because of their "lack of financial responsibility." This was the level of destruction that the pandemic brought into the home and lives of a family.

Indeed, many people thrived, but it was also a very bold reality that many people struggled during the pandemic. I have said it multiple times, and I will probably say it again before the end of this book: No one knows what someone else is going through. That is privileged information that is only available to the person, or persons, who are stuck in that dark hole of financial disdain. This is where our emotional health and well-being are affected, and no one will know how bad it is until we speak or reach out for a lifesaver. There is always a lifesaver or destiny helper somewhere for us. They come in diverse ways.

Use the knowledge you have been given and utilize sources to help you on your road to financial freedom. Don't rush the process, and don't be impatient. I am often reminding individuals who complain about their weight-loss journey that they need to be mindful that they didn't gain weight over a couple of days. They need to be patient, be grateful for the small losses, and celebrate the accumulated losses at the end of the journey. Do the same with your finances; pay extra if you can and focus on paying off one account at a time. Guess what? I have faith in you, and I know that you can do anything you put your mind to. You can do all things through Christ, who strengthens you (Philippians 4:13).

Conclusion

We have reached the part of the book where you know that you either applaud that you've stayed awake or where you want more. This book has been brewing for a very long time, and I decided that it was time to share my unbiased opinion about COVID-19. I was filled with all kinds of emotions because I read people, and I can see (and understand) their pain points. I saw the actions and reactions of people who weren't afraid to intimidate others with their thoughts and beliefs. I had to restrain myself from saying anything because I am not, and

Chapter 7: Financial Insecurity in Your Pandemic-Altered World

will never see myself as, a superhero in a golden cape, flying around on my unicorn. My concerns are for the mental health of individuals who struggle with changes, the stresses that the pandemic unleashed on the population, and the reassurance of hope in Christ for all. It doesn't matter where in the world you are; everyone has had similar experiences. I hated to see what the callousness of bullies was doing to people who were trying to create a pandemic life while working, staying safe, and adjusting to all the sudden and constant changes.

I believe that I achieved all my goals—and more. This book is filled with real-life scenarios and stories from people who pounded the pavement from the 2020 to 2023 pandemic road. It was, and is, a very long road that we walked. We may not have felt the pains of blistered feet; we experienced a life of blisters that we had to heal so that we prevented a lifetime supply of infections. Those "infections" would be adjusting to changes, concerns about work, stress about finances, and worries about returning to work—or job hunting—as restrictions ease. We live to tell the stories of our experiences, either good or bad, and our hope for a blissful tomorrow in Christ Jesus.

No More Hiding Behind the Pandemic

Most people have learned to take the necessary precautions to stay safe. I have to say it again: The vaccine was never and is not meant to be a cure for the Coronavirus and its many variants. The vaccine was developed to build up immunity to the virus. If everyone does their part in taking precautions, this virus and its little buddies may just decide to pack up and disappear on a very angry cloud.

COVID-19 swooped in, unpacked its luggage, and took over every aspect of our lives—without having any consideration for the destruction and disruption it intended to cause. It acted like a spoiled toddler which, when it couldn't get what it wanted, unleashed different strains of the virus to hold us captive a little longer. It played a narcissistic game of chance until it realized that its days were numbered. I'm not insinuating that this pandemic is over; I am merely saying that it has realized that people are not going to stand for its bullying tactics. I have previously mentioned that the pandemic provided some positiveness. I know that a lot of people may not agree with my opinion because they saw it all as a major disruption in their not-so-perfect lives.

The pandemic came with a new set of rules that we had to learn in a short amount of time. We were forced to adjust, whether we wanted to or not. I still believe that the arrival of COVID-19 forced us to slow down. It is almost as if we ignored our mental and physical health by continuing to push ourselves until we either ended up in the hospital or on the ground, and this was nature's way of getting us to stop and listen. The only way that would happen is to stop the world in its tracks. To me, and maybe to a few others also, it was a test of our faith in Christ. We all saw the news reports about nature coming to life; fish were free to swim in peace, birds could fly around without being subjected to population, and trees and plants were thriving. For the believer, it was a call to a good fight of faith (1 Timothy 6:12). You must not grow weary of the call to which you are invited, for they who wait on the Lord at the proper time will reap a harvest; they will renew their strength (Isaiah 40: 31). I am also a firm believer that the pandemic brought families closer together, and if it didn't, it showed both parties that they needed to make the appropriate choices.

The financial side of the pandemic may have been a little crueler than was necessary, but it also taught individuals the value of

Chapter 7: Financial Insecurity in Your Pandemic-Altered World

their money. Everyone had to learn that the future may have lost its bright outlook; belts had to be tightened to curb the temptation of unnecessary spending. The last chapter presented you with a couple of good ideas and examples to re-evaluate your financial situation. The pandemic enrolled us into the School of Life—Pandemic Regulated, and we had to sign up for various courses:

- Getting to know your family.
- Learning how to save.
- Job hunting in a pandemic.
- Finding happiness amid turbulence.
- Accepting that you can't control everything in life.
- Learning to lean totally on the Lord Jesus Christ for support, strength, and providence.

This is only a very short list of all the courses that you can sign up for at the School of Life—Pandemic Regulated. The best news of all is that you didn't, and don't have to, pay for your tuition. All that you are required to do is apply everything you have learned to bring about peace, joy, and happiness in your home. It is time that we all stop using the pandemic as an excuse for our current life, work, and financial situations.

The Final Word

Thank you for joining me on this thought-provoking but very essential journey. I know that you may have a lot of pent-up emotions trapped inside of you, and you need to let them out in a respectful manner. I hope that I was able to relieve you of some of your emotions. I removed my filter and emptied about 49 percent of my pandemic-related feelings in a respectful, non-condescending manner. I don't disregard people, and I most certainly don't judge people for their beliefs.

I hope you have found this book as helpful as I intended it to be. If I may be so bold as to ask, will you please leave a review or share your pandemic coping strategies based on the topics discussed in this book? Your feedback would be greatly appreciated by me and other readers who may need a little boost in confidence.

Don't go too far because I have a second book that will be arriving hot on the heels of this one. See you soon, and until then—please make time to be kind to yourself, show compassion to others, and be an example to those who look up to you.

ABOUT THE AUTHOR

Patricia is a seasoned writer and author of several motivational and self-help books and research papers. Her key desire is to impart her readers with supportive and inspiring developmental materials that will bless and enrich their lives regardless of their ages, beliefs, or life situations.

Patricia is confident that this book will significantly help readers transition into the new era with resilience, a transformed mindset, better judgment, and improved post-pandemic life.

REFERENCES

Angshuman, and Thadoi. "25 Best Ways to Celebrate Work-Life Balance and Its Benefits." Vantage Circle, n.d. https://blog.vantagecircle.com/work-life-balance/.

"Don't Be Afraid of Change. You May Lose Something Good, but You May Gain Something Better." Tiny Buddha, n.d. https://tinybuddha.com/wisdom-quotes/dont-be-afraid-of-change-you-may-lose-something-good-but-you-may-gain-something-better/.

Axelton, Karen. "Managing Your Finances Post-COVID: Habits to Start, Keep and Drop." Experian, May 22, 2021. https://www.experian.com/blogs/ask-experian/how-to-manage-finances-post-covid/.

Barman, Jyoti Prakash. "Work from Home Setup—What Every Employee Must Have." Vantage Circle, December 16, 2022. https://blog.vantagecircle.com/work-from-home-setup.

Butler, Hazel. "The History of Remote Work: How It Became What We Know Today." Crossover, n.d. https://www.crossover.com/perspective/the-history-of-remote-work.

Coria, Rubi. "6 Ways to Make the Post-Pandemic Transition Easier on Your Finances." FINANCIAL WELLNESS CENTER, July 2, 2021. https://financialwellness.utah.edu/blog/posts/2021/julynewsletter.php.

Davis, Daniel. "5 Models for the Post-Pandemic Workplace." Harvard Business Review, July 3, 2021. https://hbr.org/2021/06/5-models-for-the-post-pandemic-workplace.

Ellin, Abby. "Special Report: How Resilience Can Get Us through the Pandemic." EverydayHealth, n.d. https://www.everydayhealth.com/wellness/state-of-resilience/.

Goodchild, Lucy. "Going Back to the Office? 6 Tips to Help You Adjust." ideas.ted.com, November 2, 2021. https://ideas.ted.com/going-back-to-the-office-6-tips-to-help-you-adjust/.

Holland, Kimberly. "The Stages of Grief: How to Understand Your Feelings." Healthline, March 5, 2021. https://www.healthline.com/health/stages-of-grief.

Horowitz, Juliana Menasce, Anna Brown, and Rachel Minkin. "A Year into the Pandemic, Long-Term Financial Impact Weighs Heavily on Many Americans." Pew Research Center, March 5, 2021. https://www.pewresearch.org/social-trends/2021/03/05/a-year-into-the-pandemic-long-term-financial-impact-weighs-heavily-on-many-americans/.

Inman, Danielle. "NRF Forecasts Retail Sales to Exceed $4.33T in 2021 as Vaccine Rollout Expands." NRF, February 24, 2021.

References

https://nrf.com/media-center/press-releases/nrf-forecasts-retail-sales-exceed-433t-2021-vaccine-rollout-expands.

Kantis, Caroline, Samantha Kiernan, Jason Socrates Bardi, Lillian Posner, and Isabella Turilli. "Updated: Timeline of the Coronavirus: Think Global Health." Think Global Health, August 18, 2023. https://www.thinkglobalhealth.org/article/updated-timeline-coronavirus.

Kashyap, Vartika. "40 Best Project Management Tools & Software for 2024." ProofHub, n.d. https://www.proofhub.com/articles/top-project-management-tools-list.

Keene, Marla. "4 Tips for Finding a Great Job after a Pandemic Gap." Vault, July 27, 2021. https://firsthand.co/blogs/job-search/how-to-find-a-great-job-after-a-pandemic-gap.

Kerr, Emma. "38 Ways to Save Money." U.S. News & World Report, March 10, 2022. https://money.usnews.com/money/personal-finance/saving-and-budgeting/slideshows/ways-to-save-money.

"How to Improve Your Financial Situation Post Covid-19." Morrows Corporate, June 8, 2021. https://www.morrows.com.au/how-to-improve-your-financial-situation-post-covid-19/.

"Mental Health and COVID-19 2021 Data." Mental Health America, n.d. https://mhanational.org/mental-health-and-covid-19-april-2022-data.

"Draconian Definition & Meaning." Merriam-Webster. Accessed March 18, 2023. https://www.merriam-webster.com/dictionary/draconian.

"Coping With Change Facing Fear and the 'New Normal.'" MindTools, n.d. https://www.mindtools.com/amgqesi/coping-with-change.

"Developing Resilience: Overcoming and Growing from Setbacks." MindTools, n.d. https://www.mindtools.com/ao310a2/developing-resilience.

Monteiro, Natasha. "10 Biggest Natural Disasters of 2020 That Shook the World Costing Money & Lives." Curly Tales, December 29, 2020. https://curlytales.com/9-natural-disasters-that-have-already-happened-in-just-5-months-of-2020/.

Pinola, Melanie. "6 Productivity Tips for Your New Hybrid Work Life." Wirecutter, July 26, 2021. https://www.nytimes.com/wirecutter/blog/productivity-tips-for-hybrid-work/.

"Post-Pandemic Anxiety: Life Is Returning to Normal, so Why Do You Feel Anxious?" Weill Cornell Medicine, June 3, 2021. https://weillcornell.org/news/post-pandemic-anxiety-life-is-returning-to-normal-so-why-do-you-feel-anxious.

Pot, Justin. "The Best Remote Access Software for 2024." PCMAG, n.d. https://www.pcmag.com/picks/the-best-remote-access-software.

"Inspirational Quotes at Brainyquote." BrainyQuote, n.d. https://www.brainyquote.com/.

"A Quote from Way of the Peaceful Warrior." Goodreads, n.d. https://www.goodreads.com/quotes/2232590-the-secret-of-change-is-to-focus-all-your-energy.

"Jodi Picoult Quote." AZ Quotes, n.d. https://www.azquotes.com/quote/386694.

References

"John F. Kennedy Quote." BrainyQuote, n.d. https://www.brainyquote.com/quotes/john_f_kennedy_121068.

"Kristin Armstrong Quote." BrainyQuote, n.d. https://www.brainyquote.com/quotes/kristin_armstrong_569029.

"R. Buckminster Fuller Quote." AZ Quotes, n.d. https://www.azquotes.com/quote/347381?ref=changes-in-society.

"Sun Tzu Quote." Goodreads, n.d. https://www.goodreads.com/quotes/659546-in-the-midst-of-chaos-there-is-also-opportunity.

Sanfilippo, Marisa. "How to Improve Your Work-Life Balance." Business News Daily, n.d. https://www.businessnewsdaily.com/5244-improve-work-life-balance-today.html.

Silver, Laura, Patrick Van Kessel, Christine Huang, and Laura Clancy. "The Pandemic and Other Difficulties." Pew Research Center, November 18, 2021. https://www.pewresearch.org/global/2021/11/18/the-pandemic-and-other-difficulties/.

"The Six Million Dollar Man." Wikipedia, n.d. https://en.wikipedia.org/w/index.php?title=The_Six_Million_Dollar_Man&oldid=1145595236.

Smith Rogers, Lindsay. "Where We Are in the Pandemic." Johns Hopkins Bloomberg School of Public Health, May 24, 2022. https://publichealth.jhu.edu/2022/where-we-are-in-the-pandemic.

"Star Trek: The Original Series." Wikipedia, n.d. https://en.wikipedia.org/wiki/Star_Trek:_The_Original_Series.

"The Pandemic Has Changed Us, Permanently." WebMD, n.d. https://www.webmd.com/special-reports/covid-second-anniversary/20220120/how-we-changed.

Taylor, Derrick Bryson. "A Timeline of the Coronavirus Pandemic." The New York Times, March 17, 2021. https://www.nytimes.com/article/coronavirus-timeline.html.

"10 Tips for Staying Productive When Working from Home: Travelers Insurance." Travelers, n.d. https://www.travelers.com/resources/home/working-remotely/10-tips-for-staying-productive-when-working-from-home.

Tymkiw, Catherine. "How Covid-19 Changed Our Saving and Spending Habits." Investopedia, n.d. https://www.investopedia.com/how-covid-19-changed-our-saving-and-spending-habits-5184327.

"Covid-19 Pandemic Triggers 25% Increase in Prevalence of Anxiety and Depression Worldwide." World Health Organization, March 2, 2022. https://www.who.int/news/item/02-03-2022-covid-19-pandemic-triggers-25-increase-in-prevalence-of-anxiety-and-depression-worldwide.

"Timeline: WHO's Covid-19 Response." World Health Organization, n.d. https://www.who.int/emergencies/diseases/novel-coronavirus-2019/interactive-timeline.

Williams, Geoff. "Tweaking Your Budget for When You Return to the Workplace." U.S. News & World Report, October 13, 2020. https://money.usnews.com/money/personal-finance/saving-and-budgeting/articles/tweaking-your-budget-when-you-return-to-the-workplace.

Printed in the USA
CPSIA information can be obtained
at www.ICGtesting.com
CBHW072031140924
14363CB00011B/303